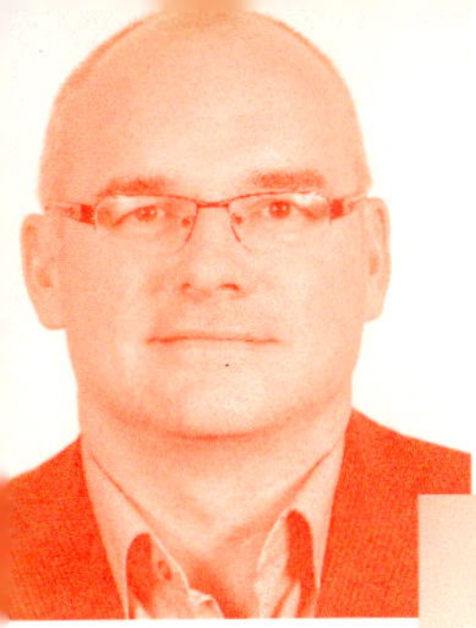
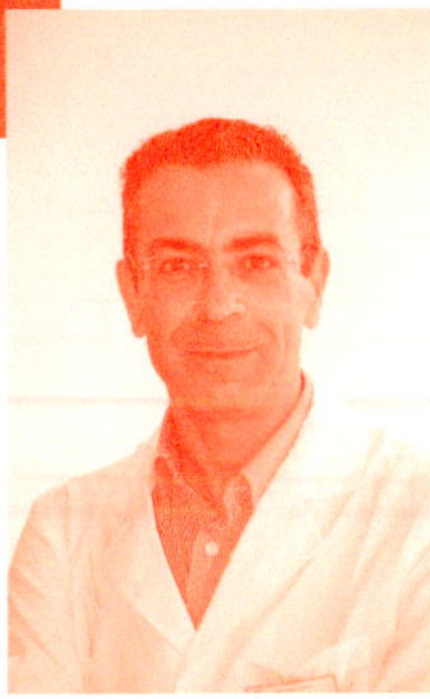
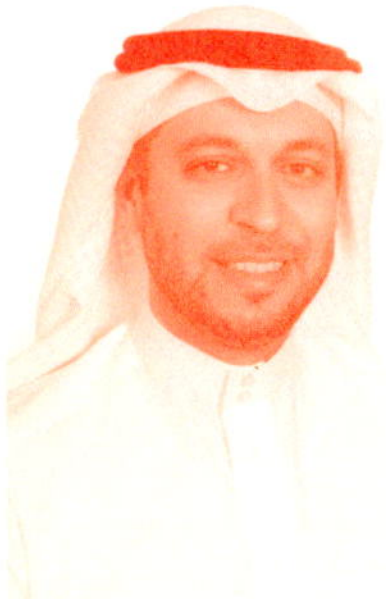
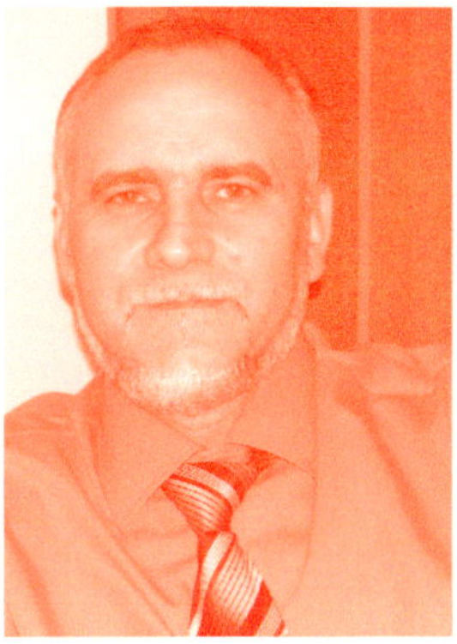
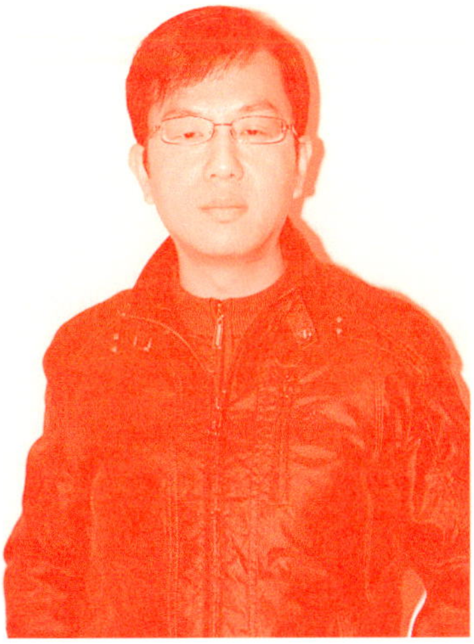
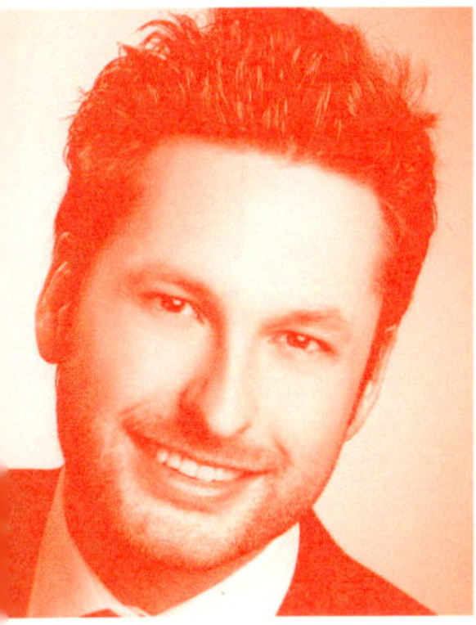
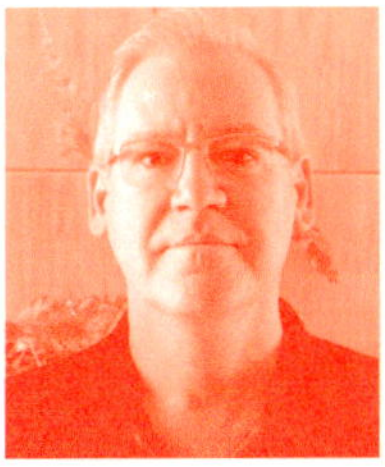

IntechOpen

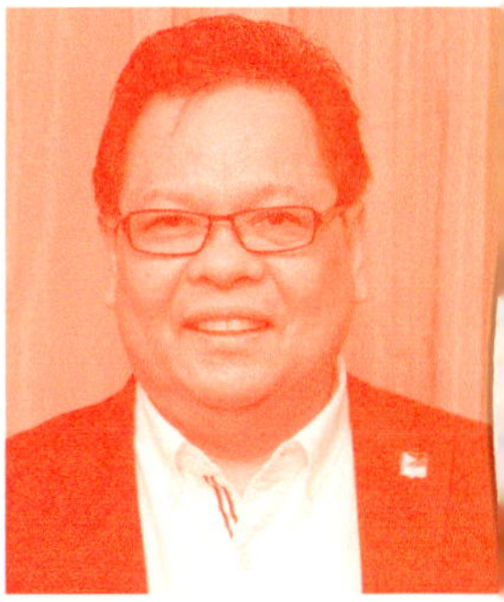
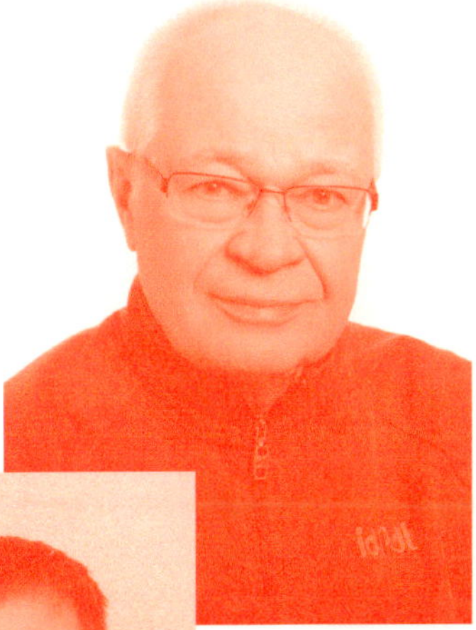
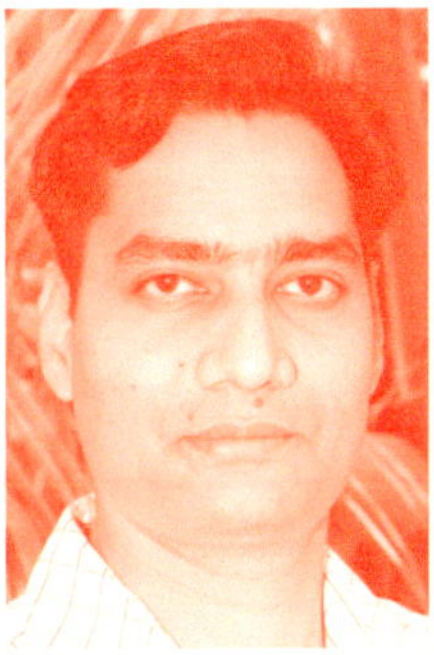
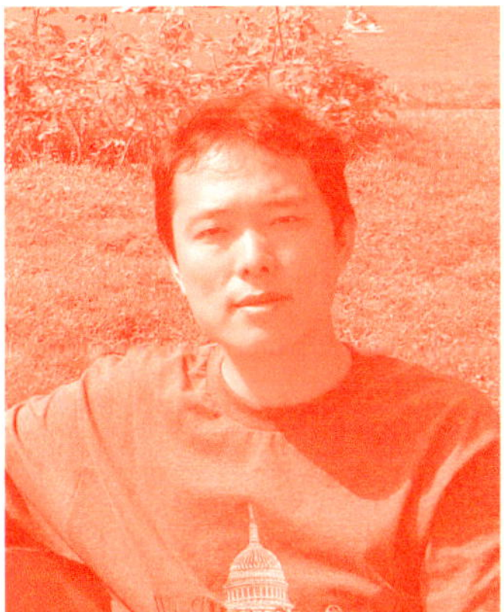
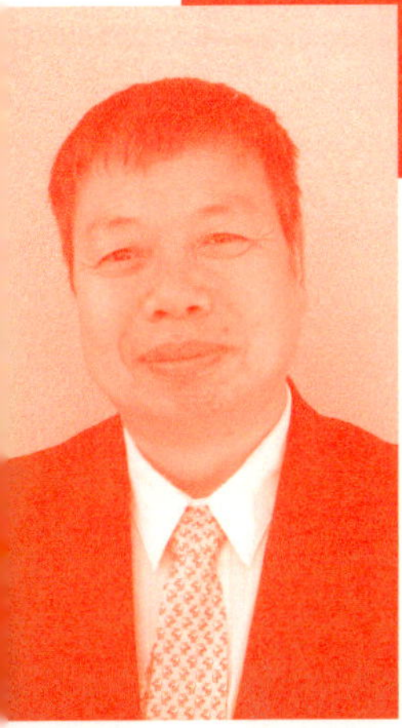
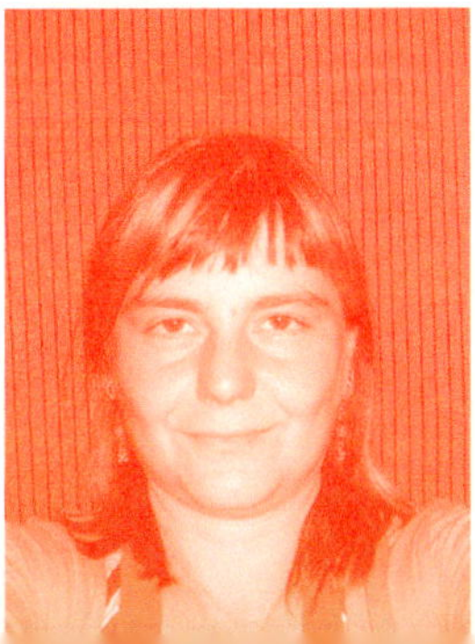

Magnetic Resonance Imaging

Edited by Lachezar Manchev

Published in London, United Kingdom

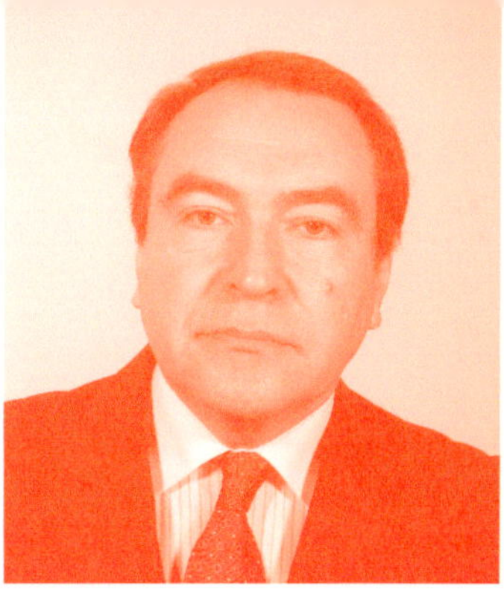
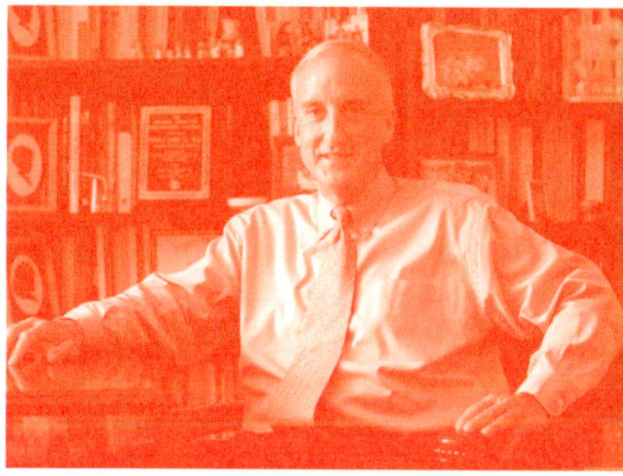
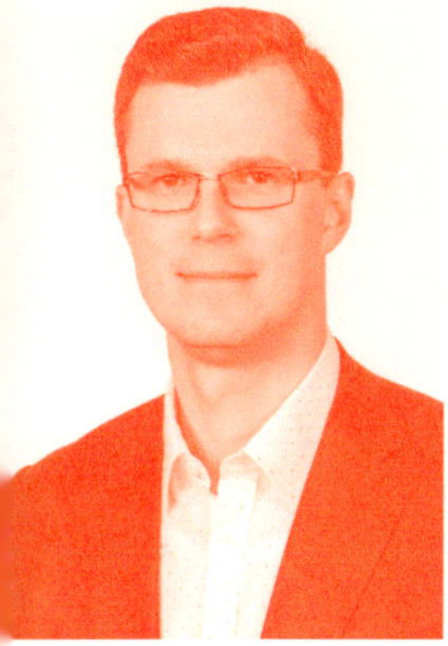
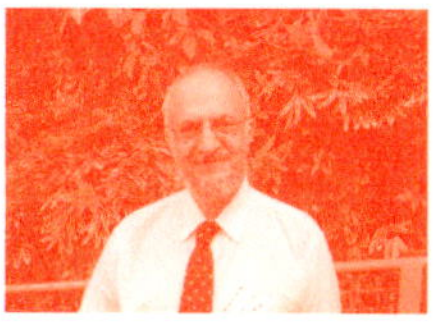
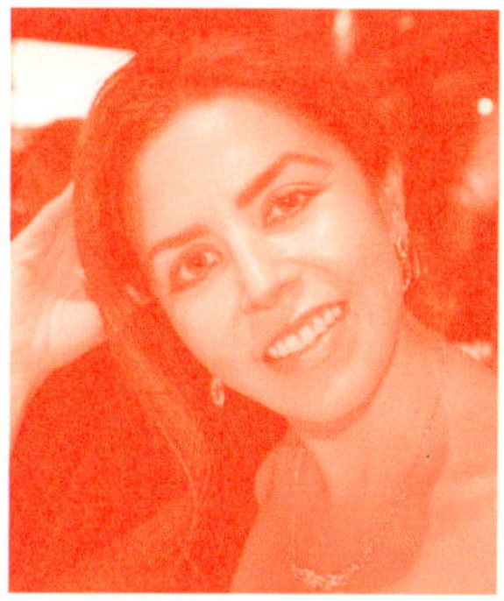

Supporting open minds since 2005

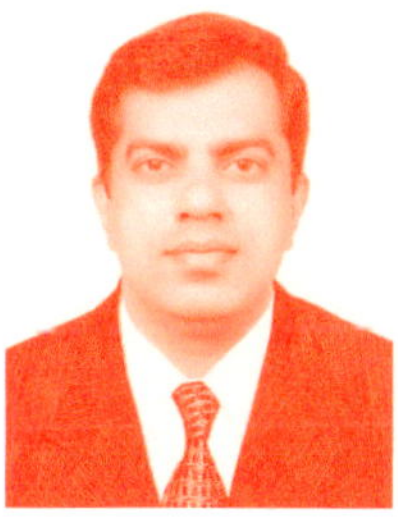
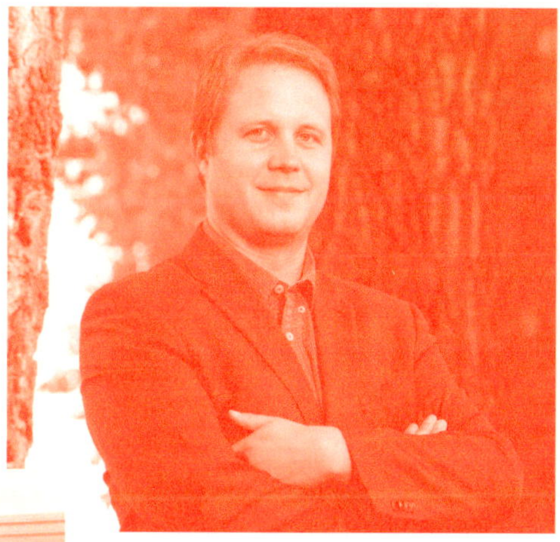
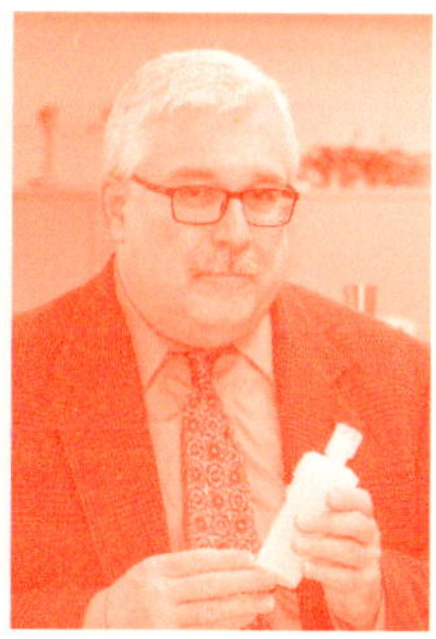
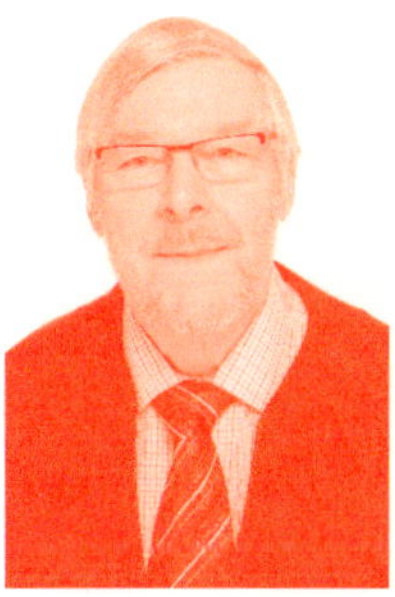
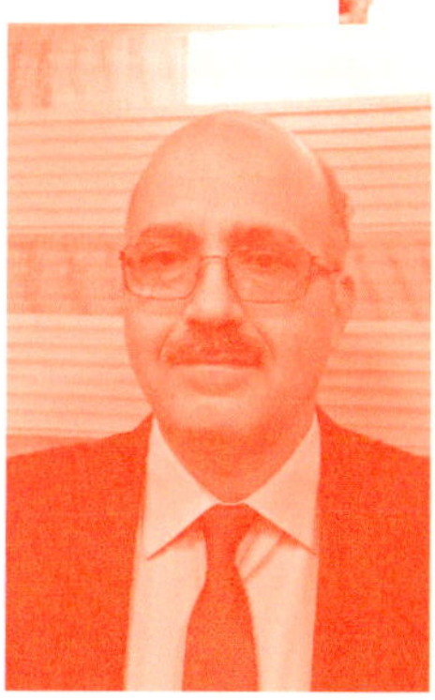
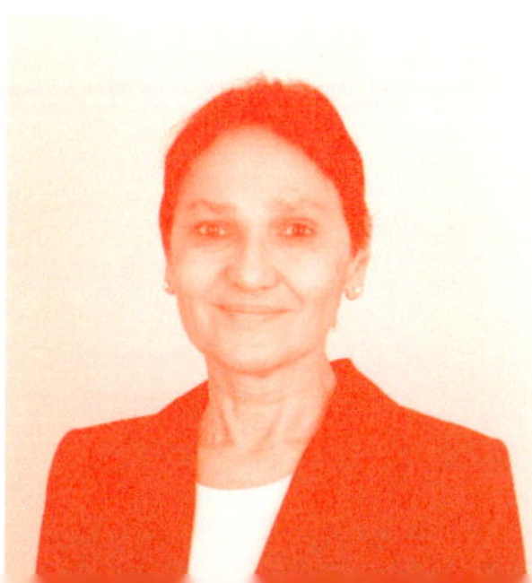
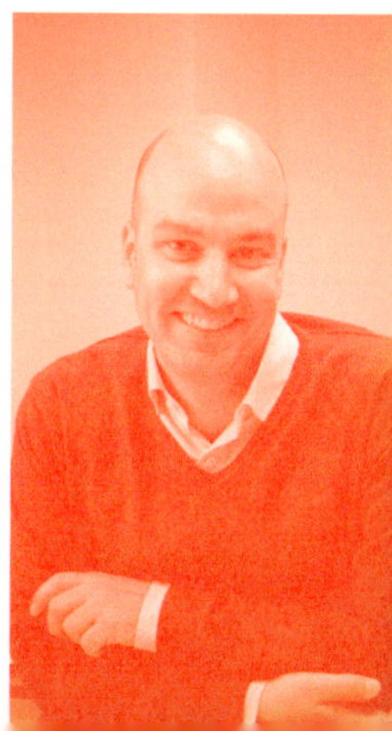

Magnetic Resonance Imaging
http://dx.doi.org/10.5772/intechopen.78456
Edited by Lachezar Manchev

Contributors
Qi Yang, Chengxi Yan, Bashar Issa, Ihab M. Obaidat, Alexei Ouriadov, Matthew Fox, Chunhao Wang, Fang-Fang Yin, Neelima Katukuri, Lachezar Manchev

First published in London, United Kingdom, 2019 by IntechOpen
IntechOpen is the global imprint of INTECHOPEN LIMITED, registered in England and Wales, registration number: 11086078, The Shard, 25th floor, 32 London Bridge Street
London, SE19SG - United Kingdom
Printed in Croatia

British Library Cataloguing-in-Publication Data
A catalogue record for this book is available from the British Library

Additional hard and PDF copies can be obtained from orders@intechopen.com

Magnetic Resonance Imaging
Edited by Lachezar Manchev
p. cm.
Print ISBN 978-1-78923-821-1
Online ISBN 978-1-78923-822-8
eBook (PDF) ISBN 978-1-83880-173-1

For EU product safety concerns:
IN TECH d.o.o., Prolaz Marije Krucifikse Kozulić 3, 51000 Rijeka, Croatia, info@intechopen.com or visit our website at intechopen.com.

Meet the editor

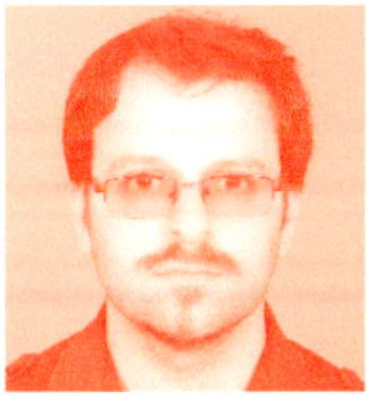

Assoc.Prof. Lachezar Ivanov Manchev, MD, PhD, graduated from the Medical Faculty at Trakia University, Stara Zagora, in 2010. Since then he has worked as a radiologist in the Department of Diagnostic Imaging at University Hospital, Stara Zagora. Between 2013 and 2018 he was an Assistant Professor in the Department of Radiology in Medical faculty, Trakia University. In 2018 he became an Associate Professor in Radiology at the same university. In his practice, Dr. Manchev presents lectures and tutorials in Bulgarian to medical, nursing, midwifery, and rehabilitation students, in subject areas including X-ray, CT, MRI, angiography, mammography, ultrasound, and DSG. Dr. Manchev also delivers lectures and tutorials in English to medical students from the United Kingdom and Republic of Ireland. Since 2016, he has worked as a part-time lecturer for the Faculty of Public Health and Health Care, University "Professor Doctor Asen Zlatarov," Burgas, Bulgaria.

Contents

Preface

Diagnostic imaging has undergone many changes over the last several years. Technical developments have defined Magnetic Resonance Imaging (MRI) as the leading diagnostic modality in different diseases. MRI is definitive and sensitive and the current requirements of medicine call for radiologists to be proficient in its use.

MRI is among the most exciting and advanced imaging modalities. Using noninvasive and invasive investigations we can visualize successfully almost all anatomical structures. MRI also has the potential to be used to assess the functions of organs and tissues.

This book provides complete and detailed information about the fast-developing field of MRI from physicians, radiologists, and other clinical specialists. It is a practical guide to using MRI in areas such as cardiology and pulmonology, among others. Chapters present scientific data that will help readers to better understand the basics of MRI and how to use it appropriately and effectively.

Lachezar Manchev, MD, PhD
Associate Professor,
Faculty of Medicine,
Trakia University,
Stara Zagora, Bulgaria

Section 1

Introduction

Chapter 1

Introductory Chapter: Magnetic Resonance Imaging in Internal Medicine

Lachezar Manchev

1. Introduction

In this book, the authors present the current trends in the development of magnetic resonance imaging (MRI) from the physical basics till the informative value in the clinical medicine. There is detailed information about the MRI in cardiovascular and pulmonary diseases, the newest contrast agents, and the relation between MRI and radiation therapy. Since its introduction due to the absence of ionizing radiation and higher sensitivity to many pathological conditions, the use of this imaging modality has increased in the recent years. The current chapter is dedicated to the role of MRI in the diagnostic medicine in general and introduction into the most significant and definitive imaging modality in the daily practice.

Magnetic resonance imaging (MRI) is a nonionizing imaging modality that uses the body's natural magnetic properties (imaging of protons) to produce detailed images with excellent anatomical details and exquisite, unmatched soft tissue contrast images from any part of the body [1].

The multiplicity of measurable MR parameters, including proton density, relaxation times, blood flow, chemical shift, diffusion, perfusion, and paramagnetic contrast agents provides unprecedented opportunities to explore morphology, pathology, physiology, and biochemistry [2].

MRI diagnoses diseases by identifying the content and distribution of hydrogen protons in the water molecules in different tissues and lesions. MRI may be effective to improve the specificity and accuracy of diagnosis and reducing the false positive rate [3].

MRI has been used in a number of nonneurologic indications, namely, spine, musculoskeletal, cardiac, hepatic, biliary, pancreatic, adrenal, renal, breast, and female pelvic imaging [4].

Cardiac magnetic resonance imaging (CMRI) is an imaging modality that can accompany the diagnostic algorithms in multiple clinical applications. It includes not only functional, but also anatomical and morphological assessments that allow ventricular and valvular functions at once to be evaluated, as well as characterization of metabolic function and perfusion. Identifications of structural assessment could be provided in multiple cardiovascular diseases like cardiomyopathies, congenital abnormalities, myocarditis, pericardial effusions, benign and malignant cardiac tumors, or congenital vascular diseases [5]. The strengths of CMR lie in its ability to comprehensively image cardiac anatomy, morphology, functions, perfusion, viability, and physiology, and the assumed information can be analyzed exactly and on time using a wide field of view of surrounding vascular and noncardiac organs [6].

The clinical indications for every MR investigations, possible pitfalls and the challenges faced in spine imaging because of anatomical and physical constraints will be discussed. The basics of advanced MRI techniques are cerebrosopinal fluid flow, diffusion, diffusion tensor imaging (DTI), dynamic contrast-enhanced T1-weighted perfusion, MR angiography, susceptibility-weighted imaging (SWI), functional imaging (fMRI), and spectroscopy [7]. Magnetic resonance imaging (MRI) plays a leading role in evaluating and detecting spinal trauma. MRI is not only a diagnostic tool in spinal trauma, but also a prognostic predictor. It is possible to predict the neurological outcome of the patients with different cord abnormalities [8].

The pulmonary MRI is also an important step in the development of the diagnostic imaging. In the past, it was taught as useless or not enough informative, because of the insufficient appearance of the lung parenchyma. In the last years, it is recommended in multiple clinical indications including the lungs, pleura, hemidiaphragms, mediastinum, etc. In addition to this, MRI is preferred because of complete absence of ionizing radiation, especially for children and young or pregnant patients.

Magnetic resonance imaging (MRI) may be considered as the preferential imaging study in specific clinical conditions like cystic fibrosis and acute pulmonary embolism, because of additional functional information on respiratory functions and regional lung perfusion [9]. At the same time, the image resolution of MRI is superior than thin-slices MDCT. So, MRI plays an important role for functional imaging in patients with interstitial and bronchial lung diseases. The capability of MRI to distinguish and describe different inflammatory pulmonary conditions using different tissue signal weighting could be used in the planning of the treatment.

Functional MRI allows measurements of perfusion, blood flow, ventilation, gas exchange as well as respiratory motion and mechanics. This could be explained with the nonionizing nature of the imaging modality, which enables regular surveillance in order to monitor therapy during clinical trials or a daily clinical practice [10].

The MRI of the chest offers a noninvasive possibility to characterize mediastinal lesions, especially according to their etiology and the involvement of surrounding tissues and organs. The intravenous administration contrast mediums provide more information than CT in tissue characterization [11].

The introduction and the use of these diagnostic modalities in a multiparametric fashion enables to better characterize mediastinal structures, for example, thymic epithelial tumors, accurate assessment of the invasion of adjacent organs and also it is extremely sensitive in the differential diagnosis of pathologic lymph nodes and metastasis [12].

Breast MRI is a modality that is progressively integrated into the daily clinical practice. Diagnostic criteria are mainly based on the American College of Radiology's BI-RADS magnetic resonance imaging categories [13]. Breast MRI is an important new study in the diagnostic algorithms for the detection and reporting of breast carcinoma. Understanding the evidence-supported benefits and potential harms of breast MRI is important to ensure the appropriate utilization of this medical resource [14].

Another important use with increased informative value in the recent years is abdomen MRI, especially in oncology, where the patients have unique challenges and opportunities. The detection and characterization of a focal liver lesion require a difference in signal intensity between the lesion and the adjacent liver parenchyma. The administration of contrast mediums is very important to accentuate the inherent differences in liver-lesion signal intensity [15].

Traditionally, T2-weighted MRI sequences are commonly used to provide structural information on the anatomy of the pancreatic ductal system and lesions. MR cholangiopancreatography (MRCP) that use heavy T2-weighted sequences has been widely applied as noninvasive alternative to endoscopic retrograde cholangiopancreatography (ERCP) for biliopancreatic duct system evaluation [16].

Magnetic resonance imaging techniques are increasingly performed to evaluate renal function and injury. These include perfusion, diffusion, and blood oxygenation level-dependent (BOLD) imaging [1–3]. Because functional, molecular, and cellular changes precede anatomic changes, functional MR imaging enables the early detection of renal disease as well as improved understanding of disease pathogenesis that could facilitate the development of better treatment options and improve patient prognosis [17].

Similar to CT in MRI are used 3D or 4D reconstructions in the three main planes to improve the quality of the images.

3D T2-weighted MRI is increasingly utilized for pelvic disease in both gender, including imaging of rectal cancer, prostate cancer, anorectal fistulas, etc. This relative rapid modality offers better soft-tissue visualization of the pelvic organs including lymph nodes and blood vessels, with potential for more widespread clinical use [18].

MRI has traditionally been used for neurologic indications, including brain tumors, cerebrovascular diseases (strokes), infections (encephalomyelitis), and congenital abnormalities. It has far-reaching real and possible clinical applications. Its usefulness has been best explored and realized in the central nervous system, especially the posterior fossa and brain stem, where most abnormalities are better identified than with computed tomography [19].

Magnetic resonance imaging (MRI) of brain diseases provides excellent anatomical details—location, size, distribution, signal characteristics and also reveals functional information about vascularity, brain edema, and the preserved brain tissues [20].

Significant role for the development of MRI has the use of contrast agents. It increased the quality and diagnostic capabilities.

Strategic localization of the agent can regionally change the tissue properties and result in preferential enhancement. MRI is unique among diagnostic modalities because it uses more than one intrinsic property of the tissue being imaged. Gadolinium-based MRI contrast agents alter one or more of their physicochemical properties dynamically when interacting with their surrounding tissues environment [21].

The current trends in MRI also include the use of nanoparticles as contrast agents. Multiple nanoparticles and complexes have been studied as MRI contrast mediums, and several formulations have been approved for clinical use in the practice and clinical trials. These contrast agents are formed either of transition and lanthanide metals or of iron oxide nanoparticles and ferrite nanoparticles. MLPs can be carefully manipulated in their composition to incorporate cationic lipids, fluorescent-lipid conjugates, targeting ligands, drugs, and PEG, containing all in a single nanosystem [22].

The last chapter of the book is dedicated to the relation between MRI and the radiation therapy. It assists successfully the detection of the exact diagnosis and could be in many cases the definitive modality for the planning of radiation therapy procedures.

Magnetic resonance imaging provides unique advantages in comparison with computed tomography (CT): added contrast information that can improve segmentation of the areas of interest, motion information that can help to better target and deliver radiation therapy, and posttreatment outcome analysis to better understand the biologic effect of radiation [23].

The implementation of MRI has a number of challenges with a balance achieved between optimal image quality and minimal geometric distortion. This process required close collaboration between MRI radiographers and radiation therapists with their differing skill sets [24]. Nowadays in practice, there is an increase in 3D and 4D MRI techniques [25].

In conclusion, we can definitely say that the optimization and development of MRI including the widespread use of contrast agents is the main investigation for structural and functional changes in the human body. The characterization of tissues, organs, and systems can be approached by multiple ways using MRI and this imaging modality has the highest achievable resolution and informative value. In our future books, we hope to complete the current scientific information with new chapters about MRI of the abdominal organs, central and peripheral nervous system, and musculoskeletal diseases.

Author details

Lachezar Manchev
Faculty of Medicine, Trakia University, Stara Zagora, Bulgaria

*Address all correspondence to: lachezar_manchev@yahoo.it

References

[1] AlObaidy M, Busireddy K, Semelka R. Critical Observations in Radiology for Medical Students. 1st ed. Willey-Blackwell: 2015. p. 4

[2] Young I. Considerations affecting signal and contrast in MR imaging. British Medical Bulletin. 1984;**40**:139-147

[3] Zhang L, Wang C, Yan Q, et al. Diagnostic and clinical application value of magnetic resonance imaging (MRI) for progressive massive fibrosis of coal worker pneumoconiosis: Case reports. Medicine. 2017;**96**(20):6890

[4] Chen M, Whitlow S. Basic Radiology. Lange; 2011;**1**:21-22

[5] Saeed I, Longmore R. Quality Evaluation in Non-Invasive Cardiovascular Imaging. Springer; 2016. pp. 95-112

[6] Bandettini W, Arai E. Advances in clinical applications of cardiovascular magnetic resonance imaging. Heart. 2008;**94**:11

[7] Vargas M, Delattre B, Boto J, et al. Advanced magnetic resonance imaging (MRI) techniques of the spine and spinal cord in children and adults. Insights Imaging. 2018;**9**(4): 549-557

[8] Saxena S, Meena D, Khokar H, Ganeriwala A. Diagnostic and prognostic role of magnetic resonance imaging in spinal trauma, and correlation with clinical profile. International Journal of Research in Medical Sciences. 2018;**6**(7):2275-2280

[9] Biederer J, Mirsadraee S, Beer M, et al. MRI of the lung (3/3)—Current applications and future perspectives. Insights Imaging. 2012;**3**(4):373-386

[10] Wielpütz M, Kauczor H. MRI of the lung—State of the art. Diagnostic and Interventional Radiology. 2012;**18**:344-353

[11] Daye D, Ackman J. Characterization of mediastinal masses by MRI: Techniques and applications. Applied Radiology. 2017;**7**:10-21

[12] Broncano J, Alvarado-Benavides AM, Bhalla S. Role of advanced magnetic resonance imaging in the assessment of malignancies of the mediastinum. World Journal of Radiology. 2019;**11**(3):27-45

[13] Herrero J. Breast magnetic resonance imaging: State of the art and clinical applications. Radiología. 2011;**53**(1):27-38

[14] DeMartini W, Lehman C, Partridge S. Breast MRI for cancer detection and characterization: A review of evidence-based clinical applications. Academic Radiology. 2008;**15**(4):408-416

[15] Low R. Magnetic resonance imaging of the abdomen: Applications in the oncology patient. Oncology. 2000;**14**(Suppl 3):5-14

[16] Yin T, Liu Y, Peeters R, Feng Y, Ni Y. Pancreatic imaging: Current status of clinical practices and small animal studies. World Journal of Methodology. 2017;**7**(3):101-107

[17] Takahashi T, Wang F, Quarles C. Current MRI techniques for the assessment of renal disease. Current Opinion in Nephrology and Hypertension. 2015;**24**(3):217-223

[18] Lim K, Noe G, Hornsey E, et al. Clinical applications of 3D T2-weighted MRI in pelvic imaging. Abdominal Imaging. 2014;**39**(5):1052-1062

[19] Cammoun D, Davis K. Clinical applications of magnetic resonance imaging—Current status. The Western Journal of Medicine. 1985;**143**(6):793-803

[20] Rees J. Advances in magnetic resonance imaging of brain tumours. Current Opinion in Neurology. 2003;**16**(6):643-650

[21] Ibrahim M, Dublin A. Magnetic Resonance Imaging (MRI), Gadolinium. StatPearls Publishing; 2018

[22] Estelrich J, Sánchez-Martín M, Busquets M. International Journal of Nanomedicine. 2015;**10**:1727-1741

[23] Chandarana H, Wang H, Tijssen R, Das I. Emerging role of MRI in radiation therapy. Journal of Magnetic Resonance Imaging. 2018;**48**(6):1468-1478

[24] Romei C, Turturici L, Tavanti L, et al. The use of chest magnetic resonance imaging in interstitial lung disease: A systematic review. European Respiratory Review. 2018;**27**:180062

[25] Rai R, Kumar S, Batumalai V, et al. The integration of MRI in radiation therapy: Collaboration of radiographers and radiation therapists. Journal of Medical Radiation Sciences. Mar 2017;**64**(1):61-68

Section 2

Cardiovascular Magnetic Resonance Imaging

Chapter 2

Cardiovascular Magnetic Resonance Imaging: From Morphology to Function

Chengxi Yan and Qi Yang

Abstract

Cardiovascular magnetic resonance imaging (CMRI) which combines high image quality with advanced techniques to probe cardiovascular system is developing rapidly. Also, as a noninvasive imaging equipment, it has been accepted widely in clinical application. CMRI techniques produce high spatial, contrast, and temporal resolution image data for evaluation of cardiac and great vessel anatomy, coronary artery imaging, regional tissue characterization, vascular blood flow, cardiac chamber filling and contraction, and myocardial perfusion, myocardial viability. This chapter will cover the basic techniques of CMRI, practical tricks of how to perform CMRI, and clinical application in a variety of congenital heart disease, coronary artery disease, and non-ischemic heart disease, etc.

Keywords: cardiovascular magnetic resonance, morphology, ventricular function, myocardial perfusion, late gadolinium enhancement, coronary artery disease

1. Introduction

CMRI is complementary to other imaging techniques, such as echocardiography, cardiac CT, and nuclear medicine. The technique has a key role in evidence-based diagnostic and therapeutic pathways in cardiovascular disease. In the past 10 years, the development of CMRI is an active field of research and continues to see a rapid expansion of new and emerging techniques. CMRI applications include assessment of myocardial ischemia and viability, cardiomyopathies, myocarditis, vascular diseases, and congenital heart disease [1].

2. Technical consideration for CMRI

CMRI uses the same basic principles of image acquisition and reconstruction as other MRI techniques. Imaging of the cardiovascular system is usually performed with cardiac gating using an adaptation of electrocardiograph gating (ECG). ECG signal is used to either prospectively trigger data acquisition or retrospectively gate data reconstruction. Respiratory gating techniques have also been utilized to compensate respiratory motion. This can be implemented with either acquisition during a consistent part of the respiratory phase (typically the end-expiratory phase) or post-processing of continuously acquired data [2].

2.1 Evaluation of cardiac morphology

Dark-blood fast spin echo is usually applied for the observation of cardiac anatomy. Another advantage of cardiac MRI is that blood can also become bright when using gradient echo sequence, such as SSFP. By using one RF pulse to generate the signal, gradient echo sequence avoids the washout effect and the signal from flowing blood appears apparently bright. Contrast between the blood and the myocardium can be generated without contrast agent [3].

The evaluation of cardiac morphology usually starts from three basic planes: axial, coronal, and sagittal planes like standard views of the thorax. **Figure 1** illustrates the standard cardiac imaging views.

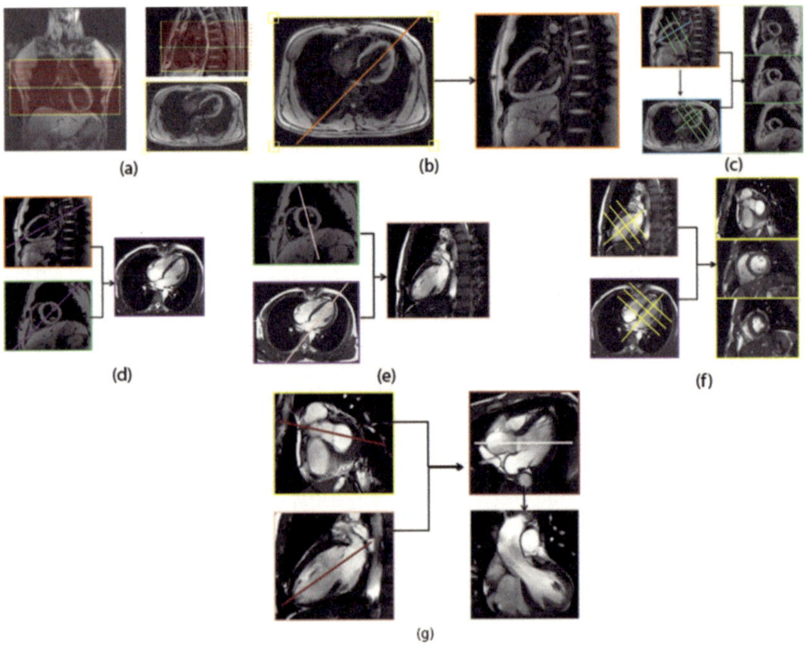

Figure 1.
Basic CMRI views. A. Localizer scans showed three standard coronal, sagittal, and transverse planes. B. Planning of the vertical long axis (VLA) image from the trans-axial image (orange line). C. Planning of the helical long axis (HLA) from VLA (blue line). Short axis (SA) images from VLA and HLA images (green line). D. Planning of 4-chamber (4-ch) image from VLA and SA images (purple line). E. Planning of 2-ch image form 4-ch image and SA image (pink line). F. SA image was obtained from 4-ch and 2-ch image (yellow line). G. Left ventricular out flow (LVOT) view from SA image and 2-ch image (brown line), and LVOT coronal view from the original LVOT image (white line).

2.2 Assessment of ventricular function

The standard approach to measure LV volume and function includes steady-state free precession (SSFP) gradient echo sequence, with one slice acquired during a breath hold of about 10–15 heartbeats [4]. It acquires in two-chamber view, four-chamber view, short-axis view, and left ventricle/right ventricular inlet-outlet view which also allow evaluation of the valvular insufficiency, outflow tract obstruction, mobility of the cardiac tumors. CMRI is the reference standard for the assessment of cardiac structure and function and is valuable for diagnosis and surgical planning in congenital heart disease. Since the sequence are vulnerable to magnetic susceptibility artifact at 3.0 T, spoiled gradient recalled echo can be used as a substitute. By tracing the endocardial and epicardial borders at end-diastole and end-systole from short-axis images occupying the heart from base to apex throughout the cardiac cycle, the parameters such as LV and RV mass, volumes, wall thickness, wall motion and ejection fraction are obtained and quantified through multiple breath hold [5].

A useful variant of cine imaging for use with motion evaluation is to combine it with magnetization tagging. These tag lines provide 3D analysis of cardiac rotation, strain, displacement, and deformation of different myocardial layers during a cardiac cycle.

2.3 Myocardial perfusion

The fundamental principle of first-pass perfusion imaging is relatively simple. Multiple imaging planes through the heart are taken every heartbeat. These images are used to track an intravenous bolus of contrast dynamically as it courses through the cardiac chambers and into the myocardium. Because the gadolinium primarily shortens T1 relaxation, the heart appears dark until contrast is delivered via blood flow or perfusion.

First-pass perfusion is divided into rest and stress perfusion. Rest perfusion detects myocardial perfusion deficits through first-pass kinetics of a contrast agent bolus, thus, it also named dynamic first-pass perfusion imaging. Ultrafast sequences like inversion recovery prepared fast gradient echo, interleaved gradient-echo echo-planar imaging, and saturation recovery SSFP sequence can assess signal intensity changes. Since myocardium has a relatively strong reserve capacity, perfusion deficits at rest is insensitive to myocardial ischemia. Induced by pharmaceutical agents, such as adenosine and dipyridamole, stress perfusion provokes coronary vasodilation and increases the contractile function compensated by increasing myocardial perfusion. Normal arteries can be dilated and respond to stress, whereas severely narrowed arteries limit flow, thus resulting deficits of the perfusion which may cause the wall motion abnormalities. Hence, an asymptomatic CAD can be identified by perfusion imaging through depicting perfusion defects under stress. There are different levels for the analysis of myocardial perfusion, which are qualitative, semi-quantitative, and fully quantitative evaluation. Since the dynamically acquired images include the whole information of first-pass perfusion, most clinicians used qualitative visual interpretation of clinical studies [6, 7].

2.4 Late gadolinium enhancement

Late gadolinium enhancement (LGE) image has been extensively validated in clinical studies and capable for detecting myocardial viability. By using segmented (or single shot) inversion-recovery prepared fast (or turbo) gradient sequence, combined with intravenous infusion of gadolinium-based contrast agent, LGE image can be obtained. By applying appropriate inverted time, the normal myocardial signal is null, and the difference between infarcted and normal myocardium is optimized. Myocyte degradation and membrane permeability increased contrast accumulation in acute myocardial infarction. Chronic myocardial infarction is characterized by fibrous tissue with larger interstitial space in which contrast agent accumulates [8].

2.5 Myocardial T1 and T2 mapping

Paramagnetic mapping techniques such as T1 mapping and T2 mapping offer a robust and reproducible quantitative assessment of both focal or diffuse fibrosis, edema and amyloidosis. T1 Mapping is performed with inversion recovery

(Look-Locker, MOLLI, ShMOLLI) or saturation recovery pulse technology (SASHA, SAPPHIRE) within a single breath hold. Myocardial T2 mapping is a technique used to reconstruct a parametric image based on the T2 value measured in each voxel. The accumulation of water in the myocardium is associated with different types of pathology, such as acute myocardial infarction, myocarditis and graft rejection [9–11].

2.6 Vascular imaging

CMRI can assess large and medium-sized vascular structures and are particularly useful in the pediatric population with congenital abnormalities of the aorta. Vascular imaging techniques includes non-contrast enhanced magnetic resonance angiography (NCE-MRA) and contrast enhanced-magnetic resonance angiography (CE-MRA).

2.6.1 NCE-MRA

Time of flight MRA (TOF-MRA) is a widely used technique for vascular imaging. By using a flow-related enhancement, it gives rise to bright blood contrast with very short TR spoiled gradient echo pulse sequences. Through one rapid RF pulse, the tissue of whose magnetization remains in the image slice, has become partially saturated. Thus, the flowing blood that moves into the slice has not received any previous pulses and appears bright or enhanced and tissues surrounding it appears dark. TOF-MRA has been used in noninvasive angiography of the intracranial angiography and carotid angiography.

More recently, 4D flow MRI referring to three-dimensional data acquired in a time-resolved, ECG-gated, manner with velocity encoding in all three spatial directions has appeared. In addition to the measurements of basic flow volumes and velocities, the estimation of derived hemodynamic biomarkers such as wall shear forces, pulse-wave velocity, pressure gradients, and other measures have been proposed. 4D flow imaging can be used in the clinical evaluation and management of patients with aortic disease. As an emerging tool for the comprehensive evaluation of cardiovascular hemodynamics with full volumetric coverage, 4D flow is a continuously developing field of research [12].

2.6.2 CE-MRA

Bolus injection of MRI contrast agent can increase the signal of the heart instantly, which can be used to generate image contrast between vessel and surrounding tissues. Imaging is usually performed on 3D-T1 weighted spoiled gradient-echo pulse sequence with short TR and TE. Blood was consistently hyper-intensity and background tissue was hypo-intensity on the contrary due to saturation effects, thus, a better MRA images is obtained, and by subtracting plain images before, a high quality MRA images are obtained.

Taking thoracic aorta CE-MRA for example. A 3D-T1 weighted spoiled gradient-echo pulse sequence is performed to acquire non-enhanced images (mask image); then, small dose of contrast agent (2 ml) is injected to test the time course of individual contrast kinetics. Imaging delay time can be calculated as estimated contrast travel time + Injection time/2 – Imaging time/2.

By injecting gadolinium-based agent intravenously (0.2 mmol/kg, 3 ml/s), another 3D-T1 weighted spoiled gradient-echo pulse sequence (same parameter as pre-contrast) was used. Image quality can be further improved by image subtraction, where a non-contrast ("mask") images is subtracted from each post-contrast images.

2.7 Coronary MRA

Whole heart CMRA, as a method of providing visualization of all three major coronary arteries in a single 3D volume, has been successfully introduced at 1.5 T MRI. Recently, some single and multicenter studies suggest that 1.5 T whole heart CMRA can eliminate the need for diagnostic coronary catheterization in many patients who are at risk of CAD. 3.0 T cardiovascular MR has become active for the evaluation of CAD in recent years (**Figure 2**). Contrast-enhanced coronary MRA at 3.0 T improves SNR and contrast-to-noise ratio and shows high accuracy in the detection of significant coronary artery stenosis. Both MDCT and CMRA can lumenographic information about the coronary arteries in the determination of existence and extent of CAD. Even though, the accuracy is be inferior to coronary CT angiography and spatial resolution needs a further improved, CMRA has the potential to be a valuable adjunct in cases where coronary calcification precludes adequate evaluation or iodinated contrast agents are contraindicated [13].

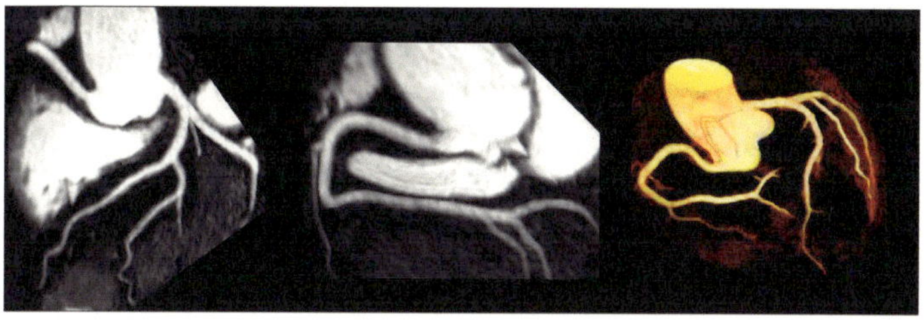

Figure 2.
3D free-breathing contrast enhancement coronary angiography at 3.0 Tesla MRI.

3. Clinical application of CMRI

3.1 Assessment of congenital heart disease

CMRI has been shown to provide helpful diagnostic information in most types of congenital heart disease. The clinical indications for a CMRI examination involve one or more of the following situations:

1. When trans-thoracic echocardiography is incapable of providing the required diagnostic information.

2. As an alternative to cardiac CT with its associated radiation in pediatric patients.

3. To obtain diagnostic information for which CMR offers unique advantages.

Detailed pre-examination planning is crucial due to the complex nature of the clinical, anatomical, and functional issues in patients with congenital heart disease. Careful review of the patient's medical history are always needed. For example, in patients with ventricular septal defect (VSD), measurement of ventricular dimensions and function is a key element of the CMRI evaluation. This can be done from the ventricular short- axis cine MRI image stack. Larger left-to-right shunts will result in left ventricular dilation but not right ventricular dilation. Quantification of the VSD shunt can be performed by calculating the Qp/Qs ratio. This can be accomplished by measuring the net blood flow in the main pulmonary artery (Qp) and the ascending aorta (Qs) using VEC MRI. VEC MRI measurements have been used to gain insight into the functional significance of an obstruction. Flow characteristics suggests a hemodynamically significant coarctation through decreased peak flow, decreased time-averaged flow, decreased acceleration rate, and prolonged deceleration with increased antegrade diastolic flow, delayed onset of descending aorta flow compared with the onset of flow in the ascending aorta [14, 15].

3.2 Assessment of CAD

CMR can provide data in all of these aspects of coronary heart disease (CAD), including cardiac morphology, global and regional myocardial function, myocardial ischemia, viability of myocardium, and the presence of coronary stenosis. Comprehensive CMRI protocols have been mainly applied to two clinical scenarios: the detection of CAD and the assessment of viability.

CMRI can accurately assess cardiac morphology, global and regional cardiac function as well as deformed ventricles. Cine imaging forms an essential component of any CMRI study in CAD. Myocardial ischemia as the principal manifestation of CAD can be detected by first-pass perfusion test. Rest myocardial blood flow will keep constant unless the significant stenosis exists, thus, physiological or pharmacological stress is necessary for the detection of myocardial ischemia. LGE images of myocardial scar using current segmented inversion recovery gradient echo pulse sequences can be obtained in one breath hold.

Gadolinium-based contrast agents are extra-cellular, thus, they can diffuse freely in to the interstitial space. In acute myocardial infarction, the cell barriers were destroyed, and distribution volume is increased. In chronic infarction myocardial cells are replaced with a fibrotic matrix which also cause the distribution volume increasing. LGE always extends from the endocardium outwards due to the process of myocyte necrosis spreading from sub-endocardium to the epicardial borders. **Figure 3** is an inversion recovery delayed-enhancement image acquisition program with phase-sensitive detection was used to acquire LGE images from an inferior non-transmural myocardial infarcted patient (yellow arrow). LGE can not only determine the presence, location and extent of infarcted myocardium, but also can identify the stunned myocardium prior to revascularization [7].

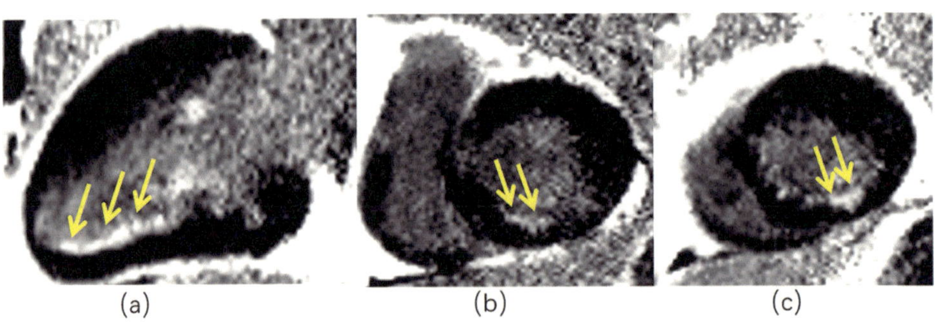

Figure 3.
An inversion recovery delayed-enhancement image acquisition program with phase-sensitive detection was used to acquire LGE images from an inferior wall non-transmural myocardial infarcted patient (yellow arrow). The inversion time (a timing option) was adjusted to null the normal myocardium. Thus, normal myocardium appears uniformly dark in these ventricular sagittal (a) and short axis (b and c) views.

3.3 Assessment of non-ischemic heart disease

Non-Ischemic heart disease includes hypertrophic cardiomyopathy (HCM), dilated cardiomyopathy (DCM), restrictive cardiomyopathy (RCM), myocarditis, et al.

Most of the non-ischemic heart disease is characterized by an alteration of ventricular and myocardial geometry or function. For the measurement of morphology and function, a stack of short-axis slices covering the entire left ventricle from the mitral plane to the apex can be used [16].

LGE further enhances the tissue characterization abilities of CMRI which shortens T1 relaxation time and brightens the area where gadolinium chelates accumulates. Myocardial tissue characterization of non-ischemic heart disease can be quantitatively evaluated through T1 mapping and T2 mapping.

3.3.1 Hypertrophic cardiomyopathy (HCM)

HCM is a genetic disease characterized by myocardial disarray, symmetrical or asymmetrical myocardial hypertrophy, most frequently occur in the septum with the loss of diastolic function or (and) possible dynamic systolic obstruction of the LV outflow tract [17]. Cine imaging can accurately assess the wall thickness, and it can be used to detect anterior motion of mitral valve leaflet in systole. Myocardial tagging imaging shows a decreasing of circumferential shortening and fractional thickening in region of thickened myocardium. LGE imaging can determine the areas of fibrosis based on increasing collagen content, which have a positive correlation with risk of lethal arrhythmias [18]. **Figure 4** is typical images of HCM diagnosed by CMR.

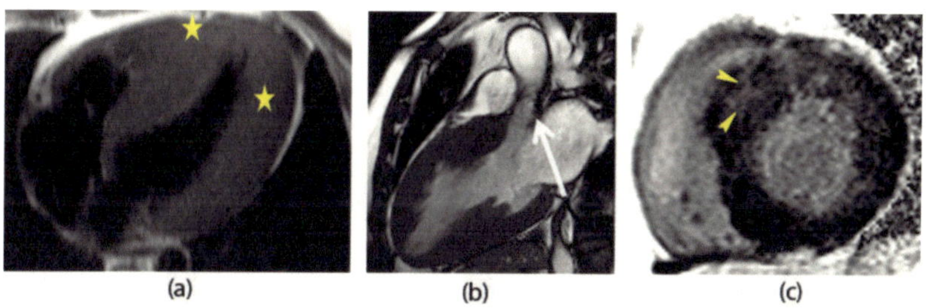

Figure 4.
Hypertrophic cardiomyopathy. A. Black blood image showed symmetric myocardial hypertrophy (yellow asterisks). B. Left ventricular outflow tract obstruction and a turbulent flow within the aorta (white arrow, B). C. LGE image demonstrated heterogeneous enhancement of the hypertrophied myocardium (yellow arrowheads).

3.3.2 Dilated cardiomyopathy (DCM)

DCM is characterized by progressive LV enlargement and deteriorated LV function with normal LV wall thickness. A diffuse myocardial fibrosis is usually detected in histopathological studies. LGE can accurately demonstrate the enhancement of ischemic DCM begins from sub-endocardial layers, while, focal fibrosis in non-ischemic DCM spares the sub-endocardial layers and shows either mid-wall patchy enhancement pattern or lack of enhancement. CMR Cine reveals an increasing LV mass, LV volume and ejection fraction as well as hypo-kinetic wall motion. Focal septal fibrosis in DCM, the so-called mid-wall sign, has been linked to ventricular arrhythmia which is a main cause of sudden death.

3.3.3 Restrictive cardiomyopathy (RCM)

Primary RCM is characterized by impaired diastolic volume of both ventricles without dysfunction of systolic, a biatrial dilation and normal or small LV size can also be detected. CMR can assess RCM accurately based on its high contrast resolution and the ability of comprehensive evaluation of cardiomyopathies. Phase contrast imaging allows quantitative assessment of flow across the atrioventricular valves. In early stage, reduced diastolic function causes the decrease of early ventricular relaxation velocities and the increase of late atrial contraction velocities. In later period, a restrictive filling will appear with rapid and tall early filling waves and much reduced atrial waves. In RCM patients, contours of ventricular cavities are maintained with atrial enlargement. Myocardial thickness is frequently increased in RCM.

3.3.4 Myocarditis

Endocardium biopsy is "golden standard" but invasive diagnosis for myocarditis. CMR is the best imaging technique to confirm suspected myocarditis and detect focal inflammation and scarring. The diagnostic criteria of CMR for myocarditis was proposed for the first time in the year of 2006 [19], which depicted that myocarditis would have the following characteristics: 1. hyper-enhancement on LGE images, not confined to specific coronary territory, but in typically sub-epicardiac or intramural (**Figure** 5); 2. The hyper-enhancement lesions is less bright than myocardial infarction and most frequently arise in the inferolateral wall. Furthermore, T2-weighted CMR T1 mapping can detect the edema which appears local or diffusing hyper-enhancement.

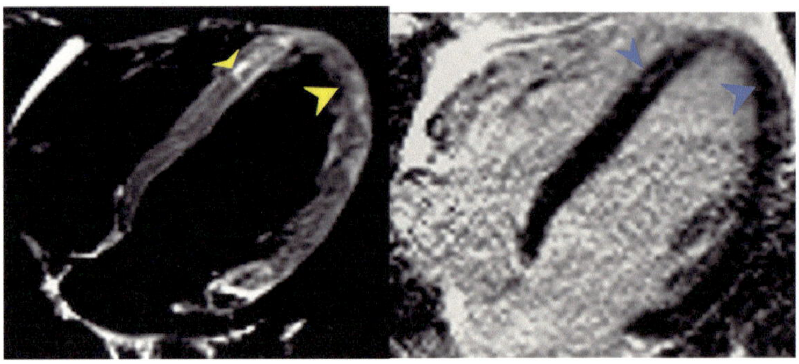

Figure 5.
A T2 Stir image from a myocarditis patient. High T2 signal indicating edema is seen in subepicardial area of septum, lateral wall, etc. (yellow arrowheads). LGE shows enhancements occur in the same area (blue arrowheads).

4. Conclusion

CMRI has revolutionized cardiac imaging. CMRI gives complementary information on LV function, perfusion, and myocardial viability. Recent advances in cardiac imaging include T1 mapping, T2 mapping, and MR-guided therapy. With the promise of higher spatial–temporal resolution and 3D coverage at higher field strength, in the near future, CMRI will become an routine tool in the diagnosis of cardiac diseases.

Conflict of interest

No conflict of interest.

DOI: http://dx.doi.org/10.5772/intechopen.84387

Author details

Chengxi Yan and Qi Yang*
Department of Radiology, Xuanwu Hospital, Capital Medical University, Beijing, China

*Address all correspondence to: yangyangqiqi@gmail.com

References

[1] von Knobelsdorff-Brenkenhoff F, Schulz-Menger J. Role of cardiovascular magnetic resonance in the guidelines of the European Society of Cardiology. Journal of Cardiovascular Magnetic Resonance. 2015;**18**. DOI: 10.1186/s12968-016-0225-6

[2] Turkbey EB, Dombroski DA. Cardiac magnetic resonance imaging: Techniques and clinical applications. Seminars in Roentgenology. 2009;**44**:67-83. DOI: 10.1053/j.ro.2008.12.001

[3] Chahal H, McClelland RL, Tandri H, Jain A, Turkbey EB, Hundley WG, et al. Obesity and right ventricular structure and function: The MESA-Right Ventricle Study. Chest. 2012;**141**:388-395. DOI: 10.1378/chest.11-0172

[4] Hundley WG, Bluemke DA, Finn JP. ACCF/ACR/AHA/NASCI/SCMR 2010 Expert Consensus Document on Cardiovascular Magnetic Resonance. Journal of the American College of Cardiology. 2010;**55**:2614-2662. DOI: 10.1016/j.jacc.2009.11.011

[5] Gerber BL, Raman SV, Nayak K. Myocardial first-pass perfusion cardiovascular magnetic resonance: History, theory, and current state of the art. Journal of Cardiovascular Magnetic Resonance. 2008;**10**:18. DOI: 10.1186/1532-429X-10-18

[6] Greenwood JP, Ripley DP, Berry C. Effect of care guided by cardiovascular magnetic resonance, myocardial perfusion scintigraphy, or NICE Guidelines on Subsequent Unnecessary Angiography Rates. JAMA. 2016;**316**:1051. DOI: 10.1001/jama.2016.12680

[7] Fihn SD, Blankenship JC, Alexander KP. 2014 ACC/AHA/AATS/PCNA/SCAI/STS Focused update of the guideline for the diagnosis and management of patients with stable ischemic heart disease: A report of the American College of Cardiology/American Heart Association Task Force on Practice Guidelines, and the American Association for Thoracic Surgery, Preventive Cardiovascular Nurses Association, Society for Cardiovascular Angiography and Interventions, and Society of Thoracic Surgeons. Journal of the American College of Cardiology. 2014;**64**:1929-1949. DOI: 10.1016/j.jacc.2014.07.017

[8] Marrouche NF, Wilber D, Hindricks G. Association of atrial tissue fibrosis identified by delayed enhancement MRI and atrial fibrillation catheter ablation. Journal of the American Medical Association. 2014;**311**:498. DOI: 10.1001/jama.2014.3

[9] Hamilton JI, Jiang Y, Chen Y. MR fingerprinting for rapid quantification of myocardial T1, T2, and proton spin density. Magnetic Resonance in Medicine. 2017;77:1446-1458. DOI: 10.1002/mrm.26216

[10] Haaf P, Garg P, Messroghli DR. Cardiac T1 mapping and extracellular volume (ECV) in clinical practice: A comprehensive review. Journal of Cardiovascular Magnetic Resonance. 2017;**18**. DOI: 10.1186/s12968-016-0308-4

[11] Moon JC, Messroghli DR, Kellman P. Myocardial T1 mapping and extracellular volume quantification: a Society for Cardiovascular Magnetic Resonance (SCMR) and CMR Working Group of the European Society of Cardiology consensus statement. Journal of Cardiovascular Magnetic Resonance. 2013;**15**:92. DOI: 10.1186/1532-429X-15-92

[12] Geiger J, Rahsepar AA, Suwa K. 4D flow MRI, cardiac function, and T1-mapping: Association of

valve-mediated changes in aortic hemodynamics with left ventricular remodeling. Journal of Magnetic Resonance Imaging. 2018;**48**:121-131. DOI: 10.1002/jmri.25916

[13] Yang Q, Li K, Li D. Coronary MRA: Technical Advances and Clinical Applications. Current Cardiovascular Imaging Reports. 2011;**4**:165-170. DOI: 10.1007/s12410-010-9064-2

[14] Steffens JC, Bourne MW, Sakuma H, et al. Quantification of collateral blood flow in coarctation of the aorta by velocity encoded cine magnetic resonance imaging. Circulation. 1994;**90**:937-943. DOI: 10.1161/01.CIR.90.2.937

[15] Ridgway JP. Cardiovascular magnetic resonance physics for clinicians: Part I. Journal of Cardiovascular Magnetic Resonance. 2010;**12**:71. DOI: 10.1186/1532-429X-12-71

[16] Bellenger NG, Burgess MI, Ray SG, Lahiri A, Coats AJ, Cleland JG, et al. Comparison of left ventricular ejection fraction and volumes in heart failure by echocardiography, radionuclide ventriculography and cardiovascular magnetic resonance; are they interchangeable? European Heart Journal. 2000;**21**(16):1387-1396. DOI: 10.1053/euhj.2000.2011

[17] Moon JC. Myocardial late gadolinium enhancement cardiovascular magnetic resonance in hypertrophic cardiomyopathy caused by mutations in troponin I. Heart. 2005;**91**:1036-1040. DOI: 10.1136/hrt.2004.041384

[18] Gersh BJ, Maron BJ, Bonow RO. 2011 ACCF/AHA Guideline for the Diagnosis and Treatment of Hypertrophic Cardiomyopathy. Journal of the American College of Cardiology. 2011;**58**:e212-e260. DOI: 10.1016/j.jacc.2011.06.011

[19] Francone M, Dymarkowski S, Kalantzi M. Assessment of ventricular coupling with real-time cine MRI and its value to differentiate constrictive pericarditis from restrictive cardiomyopathy. European Radiology. 2006;**16**:944-951. DOI: 10.1007/s00330-005-0009-0

Chapter 3

Role of Cardiac MRI in Assessment of Myocardial Viability

Neelima Katukuri

Abstract

Coronary artery disease accounts for a major cause of left ventricular systolic dysfunction. Left ventricular systolic dysfunction is reversible with revascularization in cases of hibernation and stunned myocardium. Revascularization is dependent on not only the presence but also the extent of viability, and a viable myocardium is necessary for functional recovery. For the detection of viability, non-invasive imaging techniques depend on cell membrane integrity, preserved myocardial metabolism or the absence of scar tissue (gadolinium-enhanced magnetic resonance imaging) in areas of dysfunctional myocardium. The late enhancement allows for direct visualization of necrotic or scarred tissue. By measuring the transmural extent of late enhancement, the probability of mechanical improvement can precisely be given. Cardiac MR with LGE can predict recovery of left ventricular systolic function after revascularization.

Keywords: viability, myocardial ischemia, cardiac MR, coronary heart disease, late gadolinium enhancement

1. Introduction

Coronary heart disease (CHD) is the major cause of heart failure. Among patients with ischemic cardiomyopathy, the left ventricular (LV) systolic dysfunction can result from myocardial necrosis and remodeling, myocardial hibernation, or repetitive myocardial stunning. While myocardial necrosis is irreversible, systolic dysfunction resulting from hibernation and stunning are potentially reversible states of ventricular dysfunction. An estimated 20–40% of patients with chronic ischemic LV dysfunction have the potential for significant improvement in LV function after revascularization. Revascularization is dependent not only on the presence but also the extent of viability, and a critical threshold mass of viable myocardium may be necessary for functional recovery and prognostic benefit to occur from revascularization. Assessment of myocardial viability can be done by different methods cardiac MRI, PET metabolism and perfusion, Thallium 201/Tc-sestamibi SPECT imaging and low dose dobutamine echocardiogram.

Previous studies: Studies in laboratory animals have found that, independent of wall motion or infarct age, regions exhibiting gadolinium contrast enhancement at least 10 min after the infusion of gadolinium-based contrast agents coincide with regions of myocardial necrosis and irreversible myocardial injury; regions that fail to enhance are viable [1, 2].

Clinical studies have confirmed that a normal LGE pattern occurs in dysfunctional myocardium that is viable and displays improved contractile function in response to low dose (5–10 mcg/kg/min) dobutamine infusion, while central regions with enhancement where the infarct is transmural display no contractile activity in response to the dobutamine infusion. Territories that have nontransmural necrosis display a diminished contractile response to dobutamine [3]. LGE as a marker of scar closely agrees with the finding of matching defects on PET viability scanning [4].

Assessment of myocardial viability can be done by different methods cardiac MRI, PET metabolism and perfusion, Thallium 201/Tc-sestamibi SPECT imaging and low dose dobutamine echocardiogram. Each imaging modality has its own sensitivity and specificity as shown in **Table 1**.

Further support for these findings comes from a clinical study of 32 patients with a proven MI who underwent coronary angiography; LGE, performed 3 or 14 months after the MI, accurately established the presence, location, and transmural extent of healed Q wave and non-Q wave MI [5]. Large infarcts were predominantly transmural, while small infarcts were non transmural (**Table 2**). The transmural extent of infarction predicts improvement in left ventricular function. In one study of 24 patients, the extent of dysfunctional myocardium that was not infarcted or had necrosis comprising <25% of left ventricular wall thickness, as established by LGE performed within 1 week of the MI, was the best predictor of global improvement in contractility at 3 months [6].

The extent of enhancement with LGE can predict recovery of left ventricular systolic function after revascularization [7, 8]. As an example, one study of 50 patients with coronary artery disease who had left ventricular dysfunction prior to surgical or percutaneous revascularization found that 33% of myocardial segments in 80% of patients had evidence of LGE; 38% of segments had abnormal contractility [7]. After revascularization, more dysfunctional segments without LGE improved (78 versus 17% with enhancement of more than 75% of the tissue). The likelihood of improvement in regional contractility after revascularization decreased progressively as the transmural extent of LGE increased. The percentage of the left ventricle that was dysfunctional and not enhanced was significantly related to the degree of improvement in left ventricular ejection fraction.

Comparing Modalities

	Sensitivity	Specificity	PPV	NPV
CMR				
Contrast enhanced	97	68	73	93
Dobutamine stress	94	90	86	92
Total	94	87	84	87
Conventional nuclear				
^{99m}Tc-sestambi	96	55	74	80
SPECT FDG	89	86	---	---
^{201}Tl rest, reinjection	86	63	69	85
Total	89	68	73	84
Echocardiography				
DSE	76	81	66	89
DSE SRI	82	80	---	---
End-diastolic wall thickness	94	48	53	93
Total	78	78	64	90
PET				
PET-FDG[67,70,75,79-81]	89	57	73	90
Total	89	57	73	90

Table 1.
Comparing sensitivity and specificity of various imaging modalities used for assessing myocardial viability.

Cardiac Pathologies demonstrated by CMR

Ischemic cardiomyopahy typically demonstrates a subendocardial rim of enhancement which is consistent with a known coronary territory, otherwise known as an infarct. All other enhancement patterns are independent of coronary territories.

Dilated cardiomyopathy demonstrates enhancement which is typically focal and located deep within the middle layer of the myocardium, and in conjunction with a dilated ventricular cavity.

Hypertrophic cardiomyopathy also demonstrates enhancement which is typically focal, particularly near the right ventricular insertion into the septum, and in conjunction with a thickened ventricular wall.

Amyloidosis can demonstrate a variety of patterns, including a rim of circumferential subendocardial enhancement, or overall diffuse patchy enhancement throughout the entire myocardium.

Myocarditis typically demonstrates enhancement near the epicardial surface or deep within the myocardium, but rarely at the endocardial surface.

Arrhythmogenic Right Ventricular Dysplasia (ARVD) are demonstrated by fatty infiltration and delayed enhancement in the right ventricular walls and septum.

Table 2.
Various patterns of cardiac pathology demonstrated on cardiac MRI.

Because the size of LGE enhancement may decrease with time, there may be predictive value in assessing non enhanced regions of the ventricle. One study demonstrated the value of measuring the nonenhancing wall thickness to predict improvement in systolic wall thickening [9].

CMR myocardial tagging is another noninvasive method that quantifies local myocardial segment shortening throughout the left ventricular myocardium at sites across the left ventricular wall thickness [10].

1.1 Cardiomyopathy

The high spatial resolution of CMR enables accurate assessment of ventricular volumes, ventricular systolic function (ejection fraction), and myocardial mass and wall thickness. Such analysis is useful in the assessment of patients with heart failure, for the diagnostic evaluation of cardiomyopathy, for prediction of outcomes, and may frequently be the preferred diagnostic test.

1.2 Ischemic versus nonischemic cardiomyopathy

High-resolution evaluation of regional ventricular systolic function can help differentiate between ischemic and nonischemic cardiomyopathy. LGE, which identifies myocardial scar/fibrosis, can also be used to make this distinction.

LGE is present in most patients with ischemic cardiomyopathy (81–100%) compared with 12–41% in patients without significant obstructive coronary disease [10–12]. Although LGE can be seen in ischemic and nonischemic cardiomyopathies, the patterns of LGE tend to be different in the two disorders [11–13]:

Ischemic cardiomyopathy is characterized by subendocardial and/or transmural LGE.

In comparison, isolated mid-wall or epicardial enhancement is strongly suggestive of a nonischemic cardiomyopathy. Mid-wall involvement in ischemic cardiomyopathy involved segments different from those showing subendocardial LGE [11]. **Tables 2** and **3** as shown below:

In two studies, LGE similar to that in ischemic cardiomyopathy was seen in 9–13% of patients with unobstructed coronary arteries [11, 12]. A possible explanation for this finding is recanalization after an MI [12].

LGE also may be seen in hypertrophic cardiomyopathy, myocarditis, sarcoidosis, and infiltrative cardiomyopathies such as amyloidosis [13].

Although, several powerful imaging techniques can be used clinically to identify viable tissue (and to distinguish it from scar) within dysfunctional LV segments

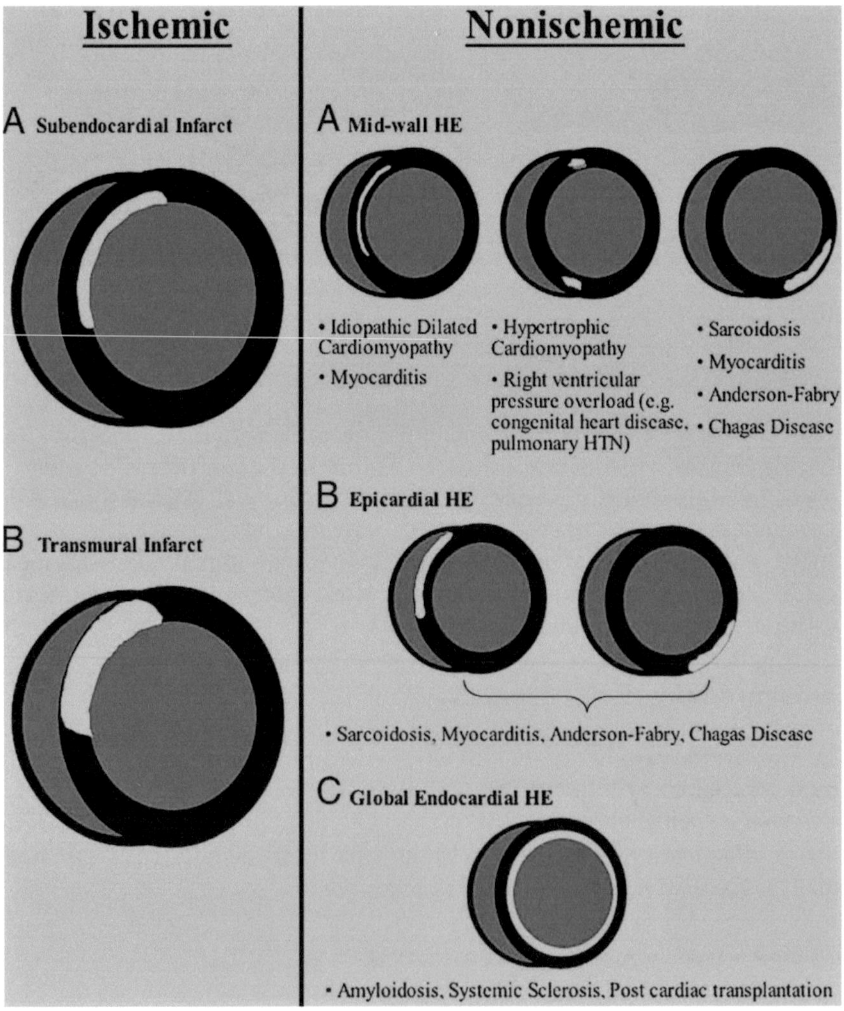

Table 3.
Differentiation of ischemic and nonischemic patterns on cardiac MRI.

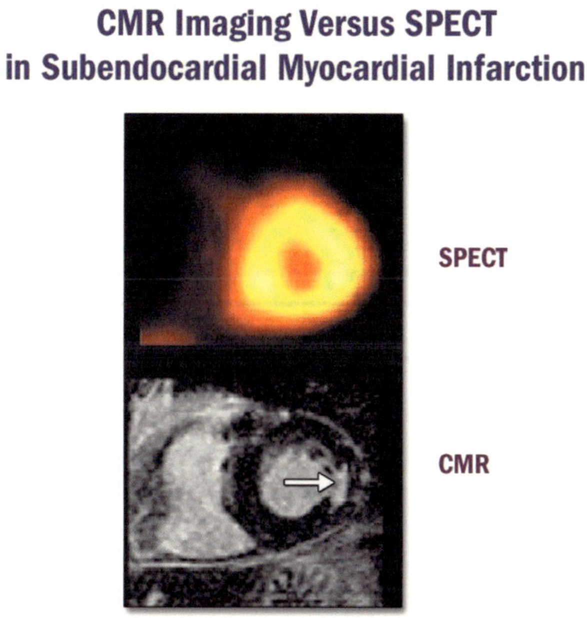

Figure 1.
Short-axis view of a patient who had an occluded left circumflex artery demonstrating normal appearing SPECT, but subendocardial myocardial infarction is easily identified on the CMR image as an area of late gadolinium enhancement in the myocardium. CMR = cardiovascular magnetic resonance; SPECT = single-photon emission computed tomography. Adapted from [14].

subtended by diseased coronary arteries. CMR has a much higher spatial resolution in detecting MI than single photon emission computed tomography (SPECT), which can miss small or localized sub endocardial infarctions (**Figure 1**). The incidental finding of late gadolinium enhancement (LGE), which reflects an area of infarcted myocardium, is independently associated with poor prognosis compared with absence of LGE. The ability to better define myocardial infarctions has led to studies to evaluate myocardial viability and recovery of wall motion after revascularization (myocardial viability). Wall segments with >50% transmural extent of infarction, the likelihood that the segment will regain function after revascularization is <8%. Wall segments with <50% transmural extent of infarction, the likelihood of the segment regaining function is much higher.

This information can be used to stratify patients more effectively and to guide their subsequent treatment. Although we still lack data from ad hoc randomized trials to prove this point unequivocally, a great number of studies in thousands of cases have provided compelling evidence that revascularization of dysfunctional but viable myocardium may lead to reverse LV remodeling and confer prognostic benefits in patients with post ischemic heart failure.

2. Conclusions

The identification of viable myocardium following an MI has important implications with regard to potential benefits following revascularization. Cardiovascular MRI provides a unique tool to assess viability as it offers superior spatial resolution and has emerged as the gold standard for the quantification of myocardial scar via LGE. The presence of viability was associated with survival benefit from coronary artery bypass graft compared with medical therapy alone in patients with severe

LV dysfunction. In the setting of complex coronary disease and concomitant LV dysfunction, a viability assessment via cardiac MRI can provide important diagnostic and prognostic information. Considering the greater spatial resolution compared with PET and the wealth of correlative pathological data, DE-MRI represents the gold standard in the detection of irreversibly damaged myocardium.

Conflict of interest

I have no 'conflict of interest' declaration.

Author details

Neelima Katukuri
University of Central Florida School of Medicine, Orlando, USA

*Address all correspondence to: pneelu@gmail.com

References

[1] Kim RJ, Fieno DS, Parrish TB, et al. Relationship of MRI delayed contrast enhancement to irreversible injury, infarct age, and contractile function. Circulation. 1999;**100**:1992

[2] Fieno DS, Kim RJ, Chen EL, et al. Contrast-enhanced magnetic resonance imaging of myocardium at risk: Distinction between reversible and irreversible injury throughout infarct healing. Journal of the American College of Cardiology. 2000;**36**:1985

[3] Gerber BL, Rochitte CE, Bluemke DA, et al. Relation between Gd-DTPA contrast enhancement and regional inotropic response in the periphery and center of myocardial infarction. Circulation. 2001;**104**:998

[4] Klein C, Nekolla SG, Bengel FM, et al. Assessment of myocardial viability with contrast-enhanced magnetic resonance imaging: Comparison with positron emission tomography. Circulation. 2002;**105**:162

[5] Wu E, Judd RM, Vargas JD, et al. Visualization of presence, location, and transmural extent of healed Q-wave and non-Q-wave myocardial infarction. Lancet. 2001;**357**:21

[6] Choi KM, Kim RJ, Gubernikoff G, et al. Transmural extent of acute myocardial infarction predicts long-term improvement in contractile function. Circulation. 2001;**104**:1101

[7] Kim RJ, Wu E, Rafael A, et al. The use of contrast-enhanced magnetic resonance imaging to identify reversible myocardial dysfunction. The New England Journal of Medicine. 2000;**343**:1445

[8] Selvanayagam JB, Kardos A, Francis JM, et al. Value of delayed-enhancement cardiovascular magnetic resonance imaging in predicting myocardial viability after surgical revascularization. Circulation. 2004;**110**:1535

[9] Ichikawa Y, Sakuma H, Suzawa N, et al. Late gadolinium-enhanced magnetic resonance imaging in acute and chronic myocardial infarction. Improved prediction of regional myocardial contraction in the chronic state by measuring thickness of non enhanced myocardium. Journal of the American College of Cardiology. 2005;**45**:901

[10] Bello D, Shah DJ, Farah GM, et al. Gadolinium cardiovascular magnetic resonance predicts reversible myocardial dysfunction and remodeling in patients with heart failure undergoing beta-blocker therapy. Circulation. 2003;**108**:1945

[11] Soriano CJ, Ridocci F, Estornell J, et al. Noninvasive diagnosis of coronary artery disease in patients with heart failure and systolic dysfunction of uncertain etiology, using late gadolinium-enhanced cardiovascular magnetic resonance. Journal of the American College of Cardiology. 2005;**45**:743

[12] McCrohon JA, Moon JC, Prasad SK, et al. Differentiation of heart failure related to dilated cardiomyopathy and coronary artery disease using gadolinium-enhanced cardiovascular magnetic resonance. Circulation. 2003;**108**:54

[13] Mahrholdt H, Wagner A, Judd RM, et al. Delayed enhancement cardiovascular magnetic resonance assessment of non-ischemic cardiomyopathies. European Heart Journal. 2005;**26**:1461

[14] Wagner A, Mahrholdt H, Holly TA, et al. Contrast-enhanced MRI and routine single photon emission computed tomography (SPECT) perfusion imaging for detection of subendocardial myocardial infarcts: An imaging study. Lancet. 2003;**361**:374-379

Section 3

Contrast Agents in Magnetic Resonance Imaging

Chapter 4

Magnetic Nanoparticles as MRI Contrast Agents

Bashar Issa and Ihab M. Obaidat

Abstract

Magnetic Resonance Imaging (MRI) is a non-invasive imaging modality that offers both anatomical and functional information. Intrinsic longitudinal and transverse relaxation times (T_1 and T_2, respectively) provide tools to manipulate image contrast. Additional control is yielded when paramagnetic and magnetic particulate materials are used as contrast materials. Superparamagnetic particles are mostly synthesized from iron oxide and are usually coated with polymers and functional particles to offer multifunctional biomedical applications. The latter include not only MRI but also cancer treatment through drug delivery and hyperthermia. This Chapter reviews the fundamental dipole–dipole diamagnetic proton relaxation mechanism dominant in water followed by a brief description of the use of gadolinium complexes as MRI contrast agent. Finally, a description of the important chemical and physical properties of magnetic nanoparticle (MNP) that define their use as MRI relaxation enhancing agents especially for T_2. The main governing models are described for the different motional regimes with few simulation results demonstrating the applicability of the given equations.

Keywords: MRI, contrast agent, nanoparticle, magnetic moment, relaxation, T_1, T_2, dipole–dipole, superparamagnetism

1. Introduction

Relaxation in Nuclear Magnetic Resonance (NMR) Spectroscopy or more relevant to this Chapter Magnetic Resonance Imaging (MRI) plays a pivotal role in the selection of experimental parameters and indeed in the image contrast. The emphasis in MRI is on longitudinal (spin–lattice) and transverse (spin–spin) relaxation times (T_1 and T_2, respectively). The advent in technology and the spread of higher field strength magnets made available a wealth of imaging pulse sequences that rely on the manipulation of T_1 and T_2 weighting to produce different diagnostic information. Early quantification of relaxation times in biological tissues hoped to find consistent differences in their values between malignant tumors and normal tissues [1]. This was based on the different abilities of water to move and sample different structural environments present due to the development of cancer. It was argued then that water content is larger in cancerous cells and water molecules are more loosely connected, however, alternative interpretations soon emerged. Nowadays various human tissues exhibit different relaxation times and it is these differences that are utilized in the wealth of experimental imaging sequences to produce different image contrast and details.

A brief introduction of MRI relaxation is given below which includes the phenomenological description, the mechanism responsible for relaxation as modulated by molecular motions before describing in more details relaxation enhancement by paramagnetic complexes. This leads the way to our main topic which is the enhancement of relaxation caused by the presence of magnetic nanoparticles (MNP).

2. Phenomenological equations of relaxation

NMR relaxation is the process by which magnetic spins return to their thermal equilibrium (Boltzmann distribution) state prior to a disturbance which is usually caused by the absorption of energy in the form of a radio frequency (RF) pulse or when the spin system is placed in a uniform magnetic field [2]. The spins return to their preferential alignment along the direction of the static magnetic field (B_0) by exchanging energy with the surrounding thermal reservoir, also known as the lattice. The latter can include spins that are physically located in the same molecule (e.g. the two hydrogen atoms in a water molecule), neighboring molecules, or solvent molecules. This process is known as spin–lattice, longitudinal or T_1 relaxation which reestablishes the state of spin polarization characterized by a net magnetization (M_0). The net magnetization depends on the strength of the magnetic field (B_0), nuclear spin (I), the gyromagnetic ratio (γ), and inversely on temperature. For a spin half ($I = ½$) system T_1 relaxation reduces the energy of the system because spins undergo a quantum transition from the high energy level to the lower one with energy difference given by the fundamental equation

$$\Delta E = h\omega_0/2\pi = \frac{\gamma h B_0}{2\pi} \tag{1}$$

Or

$$\omega_0 = \gamma B_0 \tag{2}$$

The Larmor frequency (ω_0) is the frequency of the quantized released electromagnetic energy, and h is Planck's constant. Both T_1 relaxation and the RF excitation involve the same frequency given above. The phenomenological equation describing the growth of the longitudinal magnetization M_z from the initial value $M_z(0)$ is a first order process given by (in the rotating frame)

$$\frac{dM_z}{dt} = -\frac{(M_0 - M_z)}{T_1} \tag{3}$$

with solution

$$M_z(t) = M_z(0)\exp(-t/T_1) + M_0(1 - \exp(-t/T_1)) \tag{4}$$

For liquids at room temperatures the protons relaxation times are in the range 0.1–10 s.

If the RF excitation pulse produces 90° nutation of the longitudinal magnetization, then phase coherence is established between the spins and all of them point in one direction yielding transverse magnetization M_{xy}. The lifetime of this non-zero magnetization component is characterized by a time constant referred to as spin–spin or T_2 relaxation time. Immediately after the end of the RF pulse the spins start interacting with their neighbors by exchanging energy in non-dissipative manner, unlike T_1, without net transfer to the lattice (in fact relaxation occurs during the RF pulse as well but we assume that the RF pulse duration is much shorter than T_2 relaxation). The coherence established by the RF pulse starts diminishing and the spins develop phase difference between them in the xy-plane. T_2 relaxation is related to T_1 relaxation since an increase in the longitudinal magnetization is not possible without a decrease in the transverse component, therefore, $T_2 \leq T_1$. For small molecules and large water pools that can approach bulk water T_2 values are in the range 10 ms–10 s. For solids it can be much shorter.

The phenomenological description for the transverse relaxation can also be described by a first order equation (in the rotating frame)

$$\frac{dM_{xy}}{dt} = -\frac{M_{xy}}{T_2} \tag{5}$$

leading to a solution

$$M_{xy}(t) = M_{xy}(0)\exp\left(-t/T_2\right) \tag{6}$$

This single exponential solution applies well for weak or non-interacting spins. For protons decaying in biological environments containing restrictions and molecules of various sizes the decay is non-exponential but often better described by a two exponential model reflecting compartments and exchange processes. The decay in ice is better described by a Gaussian rather than exponential process [2].

3. Relaxation mechanisms and molecular motion

Transitions between energy states, whether excitation or relaxation, are caused by oscillating magnetic fields. For resonance absorption conditions, the perturbing magnetic fields have to be oscillating at the Larmor frequency (ω_0). Other mechanisms at producing magnetic fields not only at ω_0 but also at zero and double the frequency ($2\omega_0$) will also be effective. This can be explained using arguments similar to Doppler effect [3] or more rigorously using quantum mechanics selection rules [2]. These fluctuations are produced mainly by molecular motion of the neighboring spins and by electronic excitations of paramagnetic atoms. Molecular motion modulated field fluctuations ($\vec{B}_{fluctuating}$) are dependent on the size of the nuclear spin, the environment and the presence of macromolecules, and temperature. One of the most important mechanisms is dipole–dipole interaction with a strength proportional to (μ/r^3) where μ is the magnetic moment and r is the distance between the two spins. This interaction contributes significantly to T_1 and T_2 relaxation through a distribution of molecular motional frequencies which is introduced next.

Molecules change their state of motion (typically within an average correlation time $\tau_C \sim 10^{-14}$–10^{-12} s for non-viscous fluids) due to interactions or collisions with neighboring molecules. For example, τ_C = 3.5 × 10^{-12} s for liquid water at 20° C, while it increases significantly beyond this range for solids such as ice where τ_C - 2.0 × 10^{-6} s. The frequencies describing water's state of motion will span the range 0–10^{12} Hz and, therefore, microscopic magnetic fields will be fluctuating at all these frequencies. The effect of these magnetic fields will be analogous to that of the RF pulse used in the excitation through the associated torque. Simple analysis of the cross-product equation for the torque experienced by the magnetization in the rotating frame $(\vec{B}_{fluctuating} \times \vec{M})_{rot}$ shows clearly that fluctuating magnetic field components along the x- and y-directions (i.e. high frequency components since static components in the rotating frame are actually time varying in the laboratory frame) affect both T_1 and T_2 relaxation. Components along the z-direction, however, contribute to changing transverse magnetization, i.e. T_2 processes only [4]. This is so since longitudinal field component that is static in the rotating frame is also static in the laboratory frame. These are process involve zero frequency change i.e. no net energy transfer.

When looking at the average or ensemble of molecular motion where molecules can be moving with a range of frequencies, we also need to consider the strength or equivalently the Fourier component of the motion at each particular frequency. The correlation time (τ_C) plays the role of phase memory time for which a molecule "remembers" its state of motion in a similar fashion to the role of T_2 relaxation time. The Fourier transform of the Free Induction Decay (FID) NMR signal or the decay of the transverse magnetization yields the NMR Spectrum i.e. the strength of the magnetization at a particular frequency. This leads, in a more quantitative manner, to a simple assumption about the autocorrelation function $K(\tau)$ of each magnetic field component as being a single exponential function with a time constant τ_C. [5, 6] This can be derived by considering averaging over time the product of magnetic variations ($< \Delta B_i(t)\ \Delta B_j(t) >$) experienced by hydrogen two atoms as they experience tumbling rotations in the same water molecule. This motion produces variations in the angle joining the two atoms with respect to the applied field while the inter-atomic distance does not change. Assuming that the molecules are almost spherical that undergo isotropic tumbling simplifies the analysis considerably.

For a system of short τ_C then the fast decaying $K(\tau)$ tells that molecules lose their memory of relative position to neighboring molecules quickly. The change in molecular position will be reflected in the variation of the magnetic fields both spatially and temporarily. We can consider rotational tumbling (i.e. molecular rotations enhanced by collisions or tumbling of molecules against each other and hence τ_C is the rotational correlation time) as caused by random motion. Solving the diffusion problem for a randomly rotating molecule starting from Fick's law of diffusion in spherical coordinates and introducing spherical harmonics (e.g. $Y_0 = r^{-3}(1 - 3\cos^2\vartheta)$; $Y_1 = r^{-3} sin\vartheta cos\vartheta \exp(i\varphi)$; $Y_2 = r^{-3}\sin^2\vartheta \exp(2i\varphi)$) for dipolar coupling ($\gamma^2 r^{-3}(3\cos^2\vartheta - 1)$) yields the exponential autocorrelation function [6].

$$K(\tau) = K(0)\exp(-|\tau|/\tau_C) \tag{7}$$

Fourier theory tells that the power at frequency ω, i.e. the spectral density function, is given by the Lorentzian function as follows (using a constant C)

$$J(\omega) = \frac{C\,\tau_C}{1 + \omega^2\tau_C^2} \tag{8}$$

$J(\omega)$ indicates the fraction of molecules interacting or relaxing at frequency (ω) while the constant C reflects the strength of interaction between the molecule and the lattice at frequency (ω) and is related to the mean square value of the fluctuating magnetic fields and their characteristics. For example, although the dipolar fields are the most important in inducing relaxation, they are obviously not completely random which affect the assumption ($<B_x^2> = <B_y^2> = <B_z^2> = <B^2>$).

The spectral density function for different values of the correlation time τ_C is shown below in **Figure 1**. For T_1, the height of each curve indicates the strength of coupling between the spin and the lattice at that particular frequency, and hence the efficiency of relaxation.

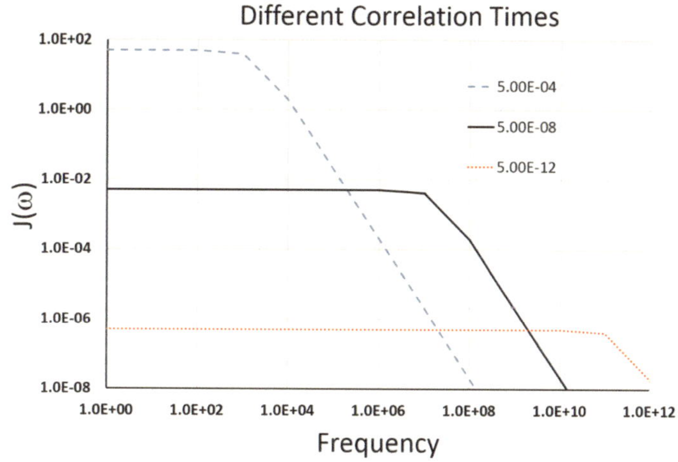

Figure 1.
The spectral density function for different values of the correlation time τ_C.

For identical spins the complete rotational relaxation rates ($1/T_1$ and $1/T_2$) induced by fluctuations at all three frequencies mentioned above (i.e. 0, ω_0, and also $2\omega_0$ where the two spins flip together) [7, 8] are given by

$$\frac{1}{T_1} = \frac{3}{10}\left(\frac{\mu_0}{4\pi}\right)^2 \frac{\gamma^4 h^2}{4\pi^2\, r^6}\left(J(\omega_0) + 4J(2\omega_0)\right) \tag{9}$$

$$= \frac{3}{10}\left(\frac{\mu_0}{4\pi}\right)^2 \frac{\gamma^4 h^2}{4\pi^2\, r^6}\left(\frac{\tau_C}{1+\omega_0^2\tau_C^2} + \frac{4\tau_C}{1+4\omega_0^2\tau_C^2}\right) \tag{10}$$

$$\frac{1}{T_2} = \frac{3}{40}\left(\frac{\mu_0}{4\pi}\right)^2 \frac{\gamma^4 h^2}{4\pi^2\, r^6}\left(3J(0) + 5J(\omega_0) + 2J(2\omega_0)\right) \tag{11}$$

$$= \frac{3}{20}\left(\frac{\mu_0}{4\pi}\right)^2 \frac{\gamma^4 h^2}{4\pi^2\, r^6}\left(3\tau_C + \frac{5\tau_C}{1+\omega_0^2\tau_C^2} + \frac{2\tau_C}{1+4\omega_0^2\tau_C^2}\right) \tag{12}$$

Different expressions are generated when considering translational motion involved in intermolecular motion with different values for the correlation times (τ_C) for both dipolar interactions and other mechanisms such as Quadrupole Relaxation, Scalar Relaxation, or Chemical Anisotropy. The equations provide asymptotic behavior for certain values of the important characteristic motional quantity ($\omega_0\tau_C$) which will be discussed later and the importance of the value $\left(\omega_0 \sim \frac{1}{\tau_C}\right)$ will be highlighted. The gyromagnetic ration (γ) points to the importance of using paramagnetic atoms (such as gadolinium and magnesium) in enhancing relaxation where the value of the electron's gyromagnetic ratio is larger than that for hydrogen by 658 times.

For example, for non-viscous liquids where the condition $\omega_0\,\tau_C \ll 1$ holds (i.e. τ_C is very small and the motion is very fast), both relaxation rates R_1 and R_2 ($R_\text{I} = 1/T_\text{i}$) are equal and are given by (for equal spin I)

$$R_1 = R_2 = \frac{2\gamma^4 h^2}{4\pi^2\, r^6}\, I(I+1)\tau_C \tag{13}$$

This regime is known as the motional averaging or extreme narrowing where relaxation is frequency independent. A brief introduction of relaxation enhancement due to the presence of paramagnetic atoms is given next in order to approach the topic of magnetic nanoparticles. The term used to describe the efficacy of CA complexes in enhancing relaxation is "relaxivity" which is defined as the relaxation rate per unit concentration of CA.

4. Proton's relaxation due to paramagnetic complexes

The use of paramagnetic centers to reduce MRI relaxation times was first reported by Bloch in 1948 [9] and has been reviewed by many workers [10, 11]. We therefore only touch upon it briefly here in order to prepare the ground for the subject of magnetic nanoparticles as MRI contrast agents (CA). The most widely used paramagnetic atom is Gd (III) with its large magnetic moment (due to the seven umpired electrons), and relatively slow electronic relaxation rate, i.e. comparable to ω_0. Relaxation due to the fluctuating magnetic fields of these electronic spins through the dipole – dipole interaction can be classified into inner- and outer–sphere relaxation mechanisms. Solvent molecules (mostly water) can be bound to the paramagnetic compound in the first or second coordination sphere (directly or indirectly through other groups, respectively). These bound water protons can exchange with other water molecules and transfer the enhanced relaxation to protons from the bulk water. Factors that influence this intramolecular interaction mechanism (i.e. inner-sphere) are the rotational correlation time for the water molecule (τ_R) which is dependent on the rotational diffusion coefficient τ_R=1/6D_R), the electronic spin relaxation time T_{1e} and T_{2e}, and the water residence correlation time τ_m (the reciprocal of the exchange rate).

For intermolecular or outer-sphere interactions then translational diffusion in the vicinity of the paramagnetic ion plays a critical role. This mechanism will dominate T_2 relaxation when discussing magnetic nanoparticles later on over that of the inner sphere. We note that the dipole–dipole interaction strength decays very fast as $1/r^6$ Eq. (13). In view of the above and based on some assumptions the expressions for T_1 and T_2 in the above equations have been modified [12] to produce the Solomon-Bloembergen-Morgan (SBM) theory for relaxation. The expressions are complicated, however, and special cases can be considered where the picture is simplified. For example, if exchange rate is either very fast or very slow then averaging relaxation rates between the bound proton pool and the bulk water protons becomes efficient or not, respectively. The former then produces one overall relaxation rate while the latter is a sum of two rates [2]. The resonant-like increase in relaxation rate seen before when $\omega_0\tau_C \sim 1$ is also present when the overall correlation rate $1/\tau_C$ approaches the Larmor frequency. This rate is now given by

$$\frac{1}{\tau_C} = \frac{1}{\tau_R} + \frac{1}{\tau_m} + \frac{1}{\tau_e} \tag{14}$$

τ_m is the residence correlation time, and τ_e is the electronic relaxation time, either T_{1e} or T_{2e}. The above discussion of paramagnetic relaxation enhancement clearly shows that there are many parameters that can be adjusted in order to adjust the inner-sphere relaxation process more than the outer-sphere one. Although, in general, both inner- and outer-processes contribute equally to overall proton relaxation, factors such as residence correlation time τ_m, hydration number, and the distance of closest approach (the smallest distance between water proton and the paramagnetic atom) can affect more the inner-sphere relaxation process. These parameters can be adjusted during the design and synthesis stages of the new contrast agent complexes in order to increase the efficiency of relaxation enhancement. For example, linking multiple Gd complexes together increases the molecular weight, hence reducing mobility and increasing rotational correlation time. Furthermore, it will increase the dipole–dipole interaction by having more paramagnetic centers. The dependence of these parameters on the applied magnetic field is also important in determining the relaxivity of these complexes [13]. We will next describe relaxation enhancement due to MNP.

5. Magnetic nanoparticles (MNP)

Nanoparticles (NP) are materials that exhibit a size (largest dimension) in the range 1 to 100 nanometers (nm) and usually contain from several hundreds to 10^5 atoms. Recent advances in material synthesis science have enabled engineers and scientist to control the size, structure, and morphology of NP to high precision in the nano-scale where the classic laws of physics are different from that at the bulk scale. As the size of the particle decreases, the ratio of the surface area to the volume of the particle increases. For nanoparticles, this ratio becomes significantly large causing a large portion of the atoms to reside on the surface compared to those in the core of the particle. For example, for a particle of 1 μm in diameter, nearly 0.15% of its atoms are on the surface, while for a particle of 6 nm in diameter nearly 20% of its atoms are on the surface [14].

Magnetic materials are those materials that show a response to an applied magnetic field. The range of applications for this type of particles is very large and still increasing as synthesis methods improve further to control the size, size distribution, stoichiometry and the surface structure of NP. Applications include biomedical [15, 16], magnetic hyperthermia [17, 18], drug and peptide delivery systems and in the diagnosis and treatment of diseases [19, 20], magnetic fluids [20], water treatment [21], magnetic information and energy storage [22]. The application of magnetic nanoparticles also highly depends on the stability of the particles particularly for biomedical applications as efforts continue to protect the particles against oxidization and corrosion. Some of these challenges can be resolved by modifying the surface of the particle by coating with organic or inorganic materials such as starch, dextran or polyethylene glycol (PEG) [23, 24]. In addition to particles synthesized out of iron oxides, natural magnetized particles were also examined (red blood cell suspensions [25] and samples of liver or ferritin) to examine the different relaxation models mentioned below.

5.1 Physical and chemical properties of MNP

For MRI application as a Contrast Agent (CA) the interest is on superparamagnetic nanoparticles with a magnetic moment that is characterized by two important properties: firstly, a paramagnetic magnetism where the magnetic moment disappears when the magnetic field is removed; and secondly, a giant or super – ferromagnetic like – moment due to the alignment of spins along the applied magnetic field. If the particle is sufficiently reduced in size, then a state of single-domain is attained and it becomes superparamagnetic. In this state, the magnetic moment of the particle behaves as that of a single atom (like a paramagnet) but with much larger magnitude. Ferrimagnetic materials (such as magnetite Fe_3O_4 and maghemite γ-Fe_2O_3) are compounds of different atoms residing on different lattice sites with antiparallel magnetic moments. In these materials, the magnetic moments do not cancel out since they have different magnitudes which results in a net spontaneous magnetic moment. When placed in a magnetic field, antiferromagnetic and ferrimagnetic materials show a behavior similar to that of ferromagnetic ones [14].

Iron has been used by many researchers to synthesize MRI CA either as iron metals [26], iron oxides [27] and ferrites substituted by other elements such as Zn, Mn, and Gd [28, 29], or indeed CA that are based on Gd or gold [30]. The addition of other elements was either to modify the magnetic moment or indeed to add another function to the CA such as heating in hyperthermia. There are many chemical and physical synthesis methods for the preparation of iron oxide nanoparticles with various degrees of control over the properties of the final product. Perhaps the most widely used method, due to its simplicity, speed, and relatively low cost, is the coprecipitation of Fe^{2+} and Fe^{3+} aqueous alkaline solutions by adding a base. The iron compounds formed by this method may have various degrees of compositions and crystal structure. The particles produced are quasi-spherical in shape, however, polydisperse in size especially if stabilizing agents such as dextran, PEG, or polysaccharides are not used. Stabilization of the ferrofluid using these agents is important in order to prevent particles from clustering. Particles tend to agglomerate in order to reduce the interfacial tension which is large due to the large surface to volume ration of nanoparticles. One of the most important characteristics of MNP (if not the most important) for medical applications is particle monodispersity. Failing to preserve monodispersity will defeat the objectives of designing and implementing any synthesis method and indeed the route of application because almost every step involved rely on the assumption of a single valued parameter rather than a range of values i.e. a distribution, at least until recently. For example, when quantifying an application of MNP a single value for each of radius, magnetization, susceptibility is given. Further difficulties ensue when clustering or agglomeration of nanoparticles exists emphasizing the importance of determining the particle radius as demonstrated by many studies such as those mentioned in ([31–33]). For MRI a more detailed study [34] of the different degrees of agglomeration induced by many types of coating concluded that clustering was the more dominant factor in changing relaxivity over other factors such as diffusion and the distance of water protons from the magnetic core.

For MRI at typical clinical magnetic fields the magnetic moment and the size of the MNP will ultimately decide the CA relaxivity and indeed its biodistribution. Therefore, it is imperative to control the aggregation of the crystals in order to define the sample size distribution. This is usually done by modifying the surface layer of the MNP, e.g. by adding some coating materials or surfactants or by changing the surface charge. Care must be exercised when doing so because the effective size or the hydrodynamic radius will also be affected. Another consequence to this will be the modification of the distance of closest approach between water protons and the MNP which reduces relaxivity. Furthermore, these mostly polymer materials will have an effective diffusion coefficient which is smaller than that of the bulk water and indeed may not have a single value across the full thickness of the coating layer. For example, we may expect the proton ability to diffuse through layers close to the metal core of the coated or aggregated MNP to be smaller than its ability in regions at the exterior regions of the coating layer close to the bulk water. Coating also leads to ambiguity in determining the magnetization, since magnetization is the magnetic moment per unit volume. The latter may not be accurately defined or indeed measurement-method dependent. Of course, further ambiguities may arise when vectorizing the coated MNP for biomedical applications such as cellular tracking and targeting in molecular imaging. The schematic given in **Figure 2** shows different possible particle geometries according to clustering and distance between different clusters within one large agglomerated coated particle.

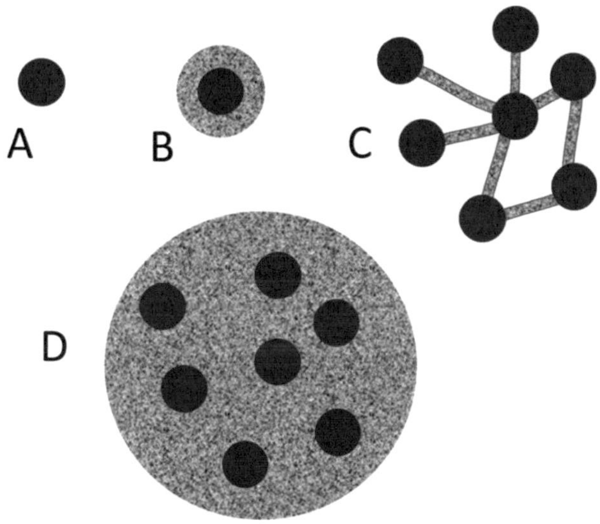

Figure 2.
Different geometries for MNP that are not agglomerated (A) uncoated; and (B) coated; while (C) connected particles (uncoated) by polymers while in D) can be considered one large agglomerated particle with a much larger hydrodynamic size due to the coating.

5.2 Proton's relaxation by MNP

Due to the ability to assemble many (e.g. 1000s) of iron atoms into the MNP the magnetic moment associated with ferro- or super-paramagnetic nanoparticles is much bigger than that associated with a single paramagnetic atom or even few linked Gd complexes. If comparable relaxation enhancement can be produced by a smaller mass of CA material, then efficiency and safety can be improved, and the amount of chemical dose administered into humans is reduced. For superparamagnetic NP the outer-sphere relaxation contribution dominates over the inner-sphere one (recall that in the paramagnetic case discussed before both mechanisms contribute comparably). Another distinction from the paramagnetic centers, is that the modulation of the dipolar interactions is provided by Néel's relaxation of the MNP (instead of the electronic relaxation) characterized by the correlation time τ_N; and possibly to a smaller extent by the Brownian relaxation characterized by the correlation time τ_D. Protons diffuse through non-fluctuating magnetic field gradients created by the mean crystal moment [35–36] which is locked along the external magnetic field. The diffusion process depends on the particle size, the solvent viscosity and temperature while the two MNP relaxation processes, depends on the size and anisotropy energy of the particle which increases exponentially with the particle volume.

Early studies of NMR relaxation as a function of field strength or frequency, known as NMR Dispersion (NMRD) curves discussed the importance of the anisotropy energy at very low fields [37]. The model successfully explained the experimental results for large superparamagnetic iron oxide (SPIO) crystals (radius ~15 nm) at high fields but failed to agree with relaxation results for smaller particles (ultra-SPIO or USPIO ~5 nm) especially in the low field range where dispersion (i.e. inflection point in the dispersion curve) in the longitudinal NMRD curves occurs [38]. For MRI at current fields [14], however, and especially at MNP typical size used in biomedical applications, Curie relaxation dominates where the NP magnet is locked along B_0 direction and the relaxation rates are then given by (under certain conditions—see next section) the following equations (similar to

Eq. (22–24) in [39]; Eq. (20) and (21) ignoring Freed's contribution in [40]; Eq. (2) and (3) in [41]):

$$\frac{1}{T_1} = \frac{32\pi}{135000}\,\frac{N_A[M]}{RD}\left(\frac{\gamma\mu_0}{4\pi}\right)^2\left\{\frac{3}{2}J_A\left(\sqrt{2\omega_I\tau_D}\right)\right\} <\mu_Z>^2 \tag{15}$$

$$\frac{1}{T_2} = \frac{32\pi}{135000}\,\frac{N_A[M]}{RD}\left(\frac{\gamma\mu_0}{4\pi}\right)^2\left\{\frac{3}{2}J_A\left(\sqrt{2\omega_I\tau_D}\right) + J_A(0)\right\} <\mu_Z>^2 \tag{16}$$

ω_I is the proton's Larmor frequency, μ_Z is the magnetic moment component along the applied field, N_A is Avogadro's number, and J_A is Ayant's density spectral function given by

$$J_A(z) = \frac{1 + 5z/8 + 5z^2/8}{1 + z + z^2 + \frac{z^3}{6} + 4z^4/81 + z^5/81 + z^6/648} \tag{17}$$

For high fields when ω_I becomes very large ($J_A(z) \rightarrow$ zero) and using the volumetric particle fraction f instead of the molar concentration $[M]$ (moles/liter) the relaxation rates can be written as

$$1/T_1 \rightarrow zero \tag{18}$$

$$1/T_2 = \frac{16}{45} f(\Delta\omega)^2\tau_D \tag{19}$$

$\Delta\omega$ is the r.m.s. Larmor frequency experienced by the proton at the surface of the particle of radius R and is given by [42, 43]

$$\Delta\omega = \sqrt{4/5}\,\mu_0 M\frac{\gamma}{3} \tag{20}$$

$\Delta\omega$ depends only on the material magnetization [43] and not the size of the particle, for example, magnetite has $\Delta\omega$ = 3.48 × 10^7 rads/s. The magnetic frequency can of course be represented in terms of the magnitude of the component of the equatorial magnetic field (B_{eq}) parallel to the external field B_0using the Larmor relationship. Magnetite's frequency will then correspond to an equatorial magnetic field B_{eq} = 1.3 kG.

5.3 Motional regimes for T$_2$

We consider in detail the effect of the diffusing motion of the water protons as they move around the MNP and sample the variations in their magnetic fields. The tortuous nature of the Brownian motion means that the water proton encounters the MNP many times in order to lose phase coherence, i.e. relax significantly or equivalently, the motion of the proton has to be very fast in order to experience and average the magnetic fields of many nanoparticles [42]. The water proton is neither confined to the magnetic field of one MNP nor is completely relaxed by diffusing around it [37]. This process defines the dynamic frequency scale or diffusional rate $\mathbf{1/\tau_D = D/d^2}$ (notice the use of "*d*", the distance of closest approach, or "*R*", the radius of the nanoparticle by many researchers). Obviously, the strength of the magnetic dephasing center has to be taken into account and this is characterized by the magnetic frequency scale which represents the efficiency by which the MNP relaxes a nearby proton as defined above in Eq. (14) [44].

The choice of the theoretical model of T_2 relaxation depends on both the size of the particles (*i.e.*, mobility) and the magnitude of the magnetic moment (*i.e.*, the dephasing effect due to field inhomogeneity) through the product parameter $\boldsymbol{\Delta\omega\ \tau_D}$. When the diffusional motion is very fast such that one MNP is unable to completely relax the protons the condition for the motional averaged regime (MAR) is fulfilled $\boldsymbol{1/\tau_D \gg \Delta\omega}$ and Eq. (19) represents the transverse relaxation rate [14].

The $1/T_2$ relaxation rate continues to increase with increasing particle size (or linearly with R^2) until reaching an asymptotic limit in $1/T_2$ (both $1/T_2$ and $1/T_2{}^*$ are equal and independent of echo time $\boldsymbol{\tau_{CP}}$ where $\boldsymbol{\tau_{CP}}$ is half the echo time for a single (Hahn) spin-echo or half the interval between successive 180° RF pulses in a CPMG sequence) when further particle size increase causes the breakdown of the MAR condition. The limited spins mobility leads to the saturation of $1/T_2{}^*$ value with further particle size increases as given by the static dephasing regime (SDR) where the protons appear less mobile, or static [43, 45, 46]. Therefore, when $\boldsymbol{\Delta\omega\ \tau_D \gg 1}$, spins relax in the magnetic field gradients created by nearby weakly or strongly magnetized particles and the diffusion coefficient becomes irrelevant. The expression for $1/T_2$ in the SDR regime is given by

$$1/_{T_2} = \frac{2\pi}{\sqrt{27}} f\ \Delta\omega \tag{21}$$

For large particles, or agglomeration of particles [47], where the refocusing RF pulses are not effective and the diffusion time $\boldsymbol{\tau_D}$ is larger than a characteristic time $\boldsymbol{\tau_L}$ given by

$$\tau_L = \left(\frac{1.49}{\Delta\omega}\right) x^{1/3}\ (1.52 + f\ x)^{5/3} \tag{22}$$

$\boldsymbol{x = \Delta\omega\ \tau_{CP}}$, the theoretical model for *T2*, known as the echo limited regime (ELR), applies and is given by

$$1/T2^{ELR} = 1.8 f\ x^{1/3}\ (1.52 + f\ x)^{5/3}/\tau_D \tag{23}$$

It should be noted that the accuracy of the above model for vary large particles is not very high and relaxation cannot just be described by a single exponential curve. This is so because dephasing is often described by a very fast component close to the surface of the particle and another slower component at farther distances.

Monte Carlo (MC) numerical simulation was used by many researchers to study T_2 relaxation [44, 48, 49] for both spherical and cylindrical particle geometry. To demonstrate the applicability of the above models we simulated transverse relaxation due to the presence of spherical MNP for both $\boldsymbol{T_2}$ and $\boldsymbol{T_2}$. We investigated relaxation under the different motional regimes and particle concentration. **Figure 3** shows $1/\boldsymbol{T_2}$ simulations for four values of the echo time $\boldsymbol{\tau_{CP}}$ ranging from 3.13×10^{-05} to 2.50×10^{-04} seconds and a volume fraction $f = 1 \times 10^{-05}$. The theoretical values for MAR and SDR are shown as well as the four curves for large particle size in the ELR regime. Available models for the latter range give an overestimate for the simulation.

Values of $1/\boldsymbol{T_2}$ simulations are shown in **Figure 4** below (for the same parameters used in **Figure 3** above). The agreement between spin-echo and gradient-echo data is evident for small particles within the MAR regime while the upper limit reached by all larger particles for all echo times is clearly demonstrated within the SDR regime consistent with Eq. (21) above.

Simulation can aid in understanding the relaxation mechanisms and developing new models by investigating the effect of different environments, particle sizes, coating types, *etc.* under both spin- and gradient-echo experimental conditions. The

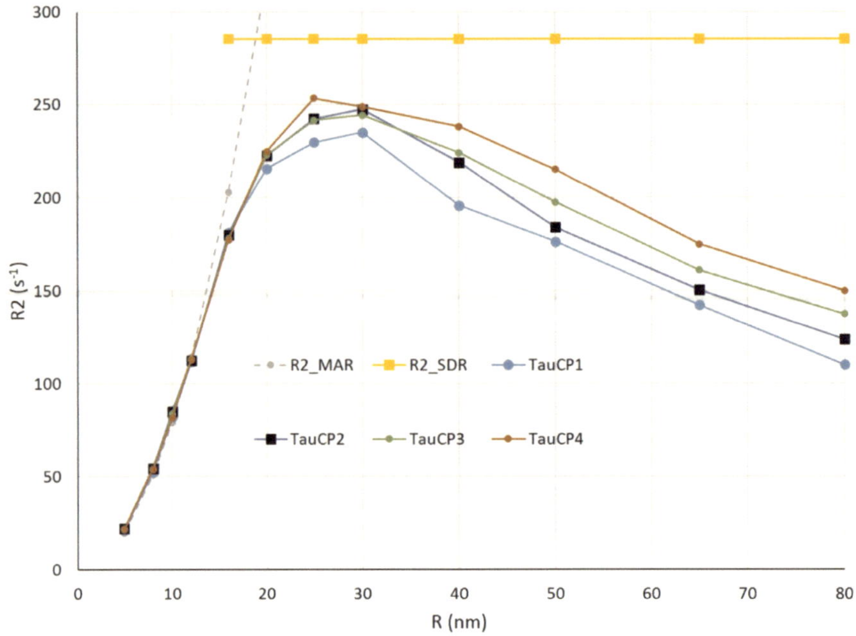

Figure 3.
$1/T_2$ simulations for four small values of the echo time τ_{CP}: 3.13×10^{-05}, 6.25×10^{-05} 1.25×10^{-04}, to 2.50×10^{-04} s. All particles used were spherical of the same size and the volume fraction $f = 1 \times 10^{-05}$.

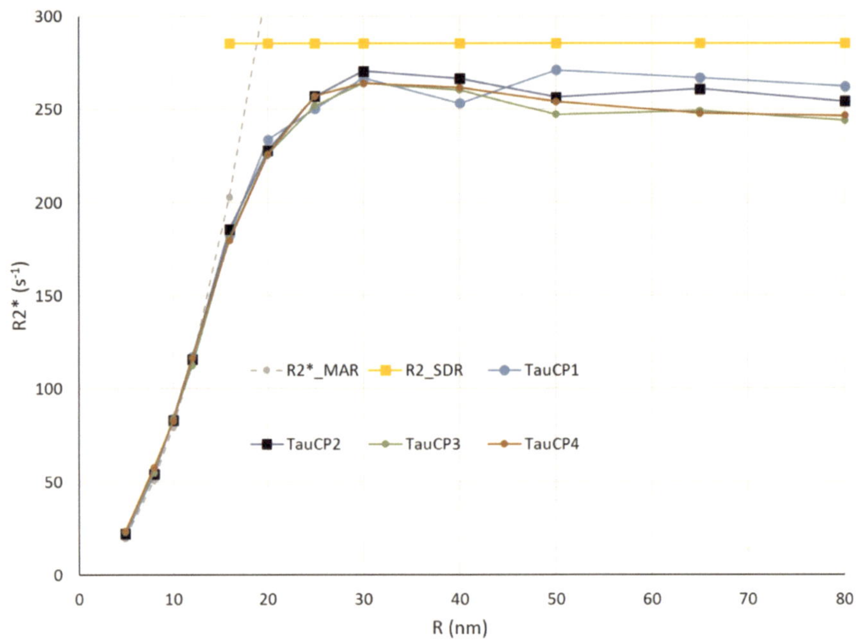

Figure 4.
$1/T_2^*$ simulations for four small values of echo time τ_{CP}: 3.13×10^{-05}, 6.25×10^{-05} 1.25×10^{-04}, to 2.50×10^{-04} s. All particles used were spherical of the same size and the volume fraction $f = 1 \times 10^{-05}$.

role of PEG coating can also be examined by specifying a regional zone around the magnetic core with a different coefficient of diffusion to that of the bulk water. Indeed, layers of coating material of different mobility can also be studied in order to simulate the environment more realistically as shown in **Figure 5**. Relaxivity was shown to decrease in [50, 51] due to increasing the water protons' distance of closest

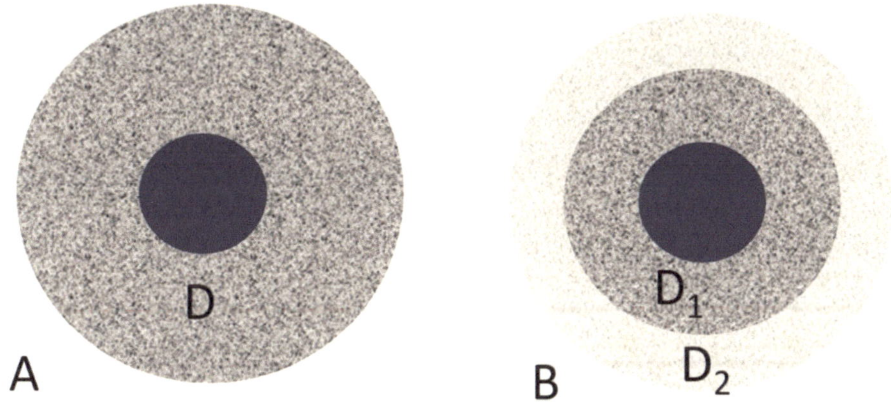

Figure 5.
Different models for the effect of the coating layer depending on the values of the diffusion coefficient according to position between the core and the bulk water. Simulations can be used to investigate the ensuing effect on relaxation.

approach by the coating layer and reduced diffusion coefficient. However, increased T_1 relaxivity was demonstrated in [51] explained by longer proton's residence time associated with the reduced diffusion coefficient.

5.4 Core-shell structures

We have seen that the magnetic moment and the size of the MNP play the most important role in determining MRI relaxivity. Therefore, it is important that the experimental determination of these quantities is accurate and independent of each other, if possible. If the sample is polydisperse, and depending on the width of the size distribution, then it may not be possible to fit the magnetization data to a single Langevin curve [52, 53]. Particle size distribution, in addition to the existence of multi-magnetization phases (e.g. more than one superparamagnetic magnetic moment component), play an important role in accurately determining the particle's magnetic moment [54]. The isolation of phases during synthesis or the existence of a dead shell layer (e.g., paramagnetic) are necessary to explain the widely reported lack of saturation of the magnetization curve even at very large applied fields [54]. A closely related topic is core-shell structures. In comparison to a single core of iron-oxide nanoparticles, core-shell structured iron/iron-oxide nanoparticles offer a much stronger T_2 shortening effect than that of iron-oxide with the same core size [55, 56]. Multifunctional NP benefit from the ability to combine iron or other metals to the conventional iron oxide material. Combined hyperthermia and MRI rely on doping iron oxide particles with metals such as Mn and Gd in order to control their thermodynamic properties [32]. Multimodality imaging offers other imaging modality in addition to MRI to help in improving the diagnostic information [56]. Recent advances in synthesis method opened the way for a better control over the particle morphology. Cubic and flower-shaped particles offer higher magnetization values through anisotropy and larger surface to volume ratios [57]. Cubic nanoparticles can have a higher degree of crystallinity and relaxivity (four times higher) than their spherical counterparts [58].

6. Conclusions

Superparamagnetic particles mostly synthesized from iron oxide exhibit large magnetic moment compared to the Gd-chelates conventionally used as MRI contrast agents. The ability to control the structure, morphology, size, and size distribution is critical to the optimum application of these magnetic nanoparticles as MRI relaxation enhancing centers. Further coating and functionalization of the surface of these particles enable their use as multifunctional particles in cancer treatment or multimodality imaging. Recent synthesis methods have produced cubic and assembled particles with improved performance in terms of larger magnetic moment which offers not only higher MRI relaxivity but also reduced dose of injected material.

Author details

Bashar Issa[1]* and Ihab M. Obaidat[2]

1 Department of Medical Diagnostic Imaging, College of Health Sciences, University of Sharjah, Sharjah, UAE

2 Department of Physics, College of Science, United Arab Emirates University, Al Ain, UAE

*Address all correspondence to: bissa@sharjah.ac.ae

References

[1] Damadian R. Tumor detection by nuclear magnetic resonance. Science. 1971;**171**(3976):1151-1153. Available from: http://www.ncbi.nlm.nih.gov/pubmed/5544870

[2] Callaghan PT. Principles of Nuclear Magnetic Resonance Microscopy. England: Oxford University Press; 1991

[3] Andrew ER. Nuclear Magnetic Resonance. Cambridge: University Press; 1955. 114 p

[4] Farrar TC, Becker ED. Pulse and Fourier Transform NMR. New york and London: Academic Press; 1971. pp. 34-45. Available from: http://www.sciencedirect.com/science/article/pii/B9780080918129500089

[5] Doob JL. The elementary Gaussian processes. Annals of Mathematical Statistics. 1944;**15**(3):229-282

[6] Levitt MH. Spin Dynamics Basics of Nuclear Magnetic Resonance. 2 ed. Chichester, England: John Wiley & Sons Ltd; 2008

[7] Solomon I. Relaxation processes in a system of two spins. Physics Review. 1955;**99**:559

[8] Lauffer RB. Paramagnetic metal complexes as water proton relaxation agents for NMR imaging: Theory and design. Chemical Reviews. 1987;**87**(5):901-927. DOI: 10.1021/cr00081a003

[9] Bloch F, Hansen WW, Packard M. The nuclear induction experiment. Physics Review. 1946;**70**:474

[10] Caravan P, Ellison JJ, McMurry TJ, Lauffer RB. Gadolinium(III) chelates as MRI contrast agents: Structure, dynamics, and applications. Chemical Reviews. 1999;**99**(9):2293-2352. DOI: 10.1021/cr980440x

[11] Sherry AD, Caravan P, Lenkinski RE. Primer on gadolinium chemistry. Journal of Magnetic Resonance Imaging. 2009;**30**(6):1240-1248

[12] Kowalewski J. In: Grant DM, Harris RK, editors. Encyclopedia of Nuclear Magnetic Resonance. Chichester: John Wiley & Sons, Ltd.; 1996. pp. 3456-3462

[13] Trattnig S, Pinker K, Ba-Ssalamah AN-HI. The optimal use of contrast agents at high field MRI. European Radiology. 2006;**16**:1280-1287

[14] Issa B, Obaidat IM, Albiss BA, Haik Y. Magnetic nanoparticles: Surface effects and properties related to biomedicine applications. International Journal of Molecular Sciences. 2013;**14**(11):21266-21305

[15] Kolhatkar AG, Jamison AC, Litvinov D, Willson RCLT. Tuning the magnetic properties of nanoparticles. International Journal of Molecular Sciences. 2013;**14**:15977-16009

[16] Lübbe AS, Bergemann C, Riess H, Lãbbe AS, Schriever F, Reichardt P, et al. Clinical experiences with magnetic drug targeting : A phase I study with 4 ′-epidoxorubicin in 14 patients with advanced solid tumors in 14 patients with advanced solid tumors. Cancer Research. 1996:4686-4693

[17] Ito A, Honda H, Kobayashi T. Cancer immunotherapy based on intracellular hyperthermia using magnetite nanoparticles: A novel concept of "heat-controlled necrosis" with heat shock protein expression. Cancer Immunology, Immunotherapy. 2006;**55**:320-328

[18] Nobuto H, Sugita T, Kubo T, Shimose S, Yasunaga Y, Murakami T, et al. Evaluation of systemic chemotherapy with magnetic liposomal doxorubicin and a dipole external

electromagnet. International Journal of Cancer. 2004;**109**(4):627-635. Available from: http://www.ncbi.nlm.nih.gov/pubmed/14991586

[19] Ruysschaert T, Paquereau L, Winterhalter M, Fournier D. Stabilization of liposomes through enzymatic polymerization of DNA. Nano Letters. 2006;**6**:2755-2757

[20] Taylor R, Coulombe S, Otanicar T, Phelan P, Gunawan A, Lv W, et al. Small particles, big impacts: A review of the diverse applications of nanofluids. Journal of Applied Physics. 2013;**113**: 011301

[21] Yavuz C, Mayo J, Yu W, Prakash A, Falkner J, Yean S, et al. Low-field magnetic separation of monodisperse Fe3O4 nanocrystals. Science (80-). 2006;**314**:964-967

[22] Singamaneni S, Bliznyuk V, Binekc C, Tsymbalc E. Magnetic nanoparticles: Recent advances in synthesis, self-assembly and applications. Journal of Materials Chemistry. 2011;**21**: 16819-16845

[23] Di Marco M, Guilbert I, Port M, Robic C, Couvreur P, Dubernet C. Colloidal stability of ultrasmall superparamagnetic iron oxide (USPIO) particles with different coatings. International Journal of Pharmaceutics. 2007;**331**:197-203

[24] Gupta AK, Gupta M. Synthesis and surface engineering of iron oxide nanoparticles for biomedical applications. Biomaterials. 2005;**26**(18): 3995-4021. Available from: http://www.ncbi.nlm.nih.gov/pubmed/15626447

[25] Lisitza N, Warren W, Song Y-Q. Study of diffusion in erythrocyte suspension using internal magnetic field inhomogeneity. Journal of Magnetic Resonance. 2007;**187**:146-154

[26] Bautista MC, Bomati-Miguel O, Zhao X, Morales MP, González-Carreño T, De Alejo RP, et al. Comparative study of ferrofluids based on dextran-coated iron oxide and metal nanoparticles for contrast agents in magnetic resonance imaging. Nanotechnology. 2004;**15**(4): S154-S159. Available from: http://stacks.iop.org/0957-4484/15/i=4/a=008?key=crossref.adfd4debc6b423edb6d2c867057ef978

[27] Elias A, Tsourkas A. Imaging circulating cells and lymphoid tissues with iron oxide nanoparticles. Hematology. 2009;**2009**:720-726

[28] Issa B, Obaidat IM, Hejasee RH, Qadri S, Haik Y. NMR relaxation in systems with magnetic nanoparticles: A temperature study. Journal of Magnetic Resonance Imaging. 2014;**39**(3):648-655

[29] Hejase H, Hayek SS, Qadri S, Haik Y. MnZnFe nanoparticles for self-controlled magnetic hyperthermia. Journal of Magnetism and Magnetic Materials. 2012;**324**(22):3620-3628. Available from: http://www.sciencedirect.com/science/article/pii/S0304885312002983

[30] Heitsch A, Smith D, Patel R, Ress D, Korgel B. Multifunctional particles: Magnetic nanocrystals and gold nanorods coated with fluorescent dye-doped silica shells. Journal of Solid State Chemistry. 2008;**181**:1590-1599

Section 4

Pulmonary Magnetic Resonance Imaging

Chapter 5

High Resolution ^{3}He Pulmonary MRI

Matthew S. Fox and Alexei V. Ouriadov

Abstract

Hyperpolarized gas MRI of the mouse lung is of great interest due to the urgent need for novel biomarkers for the assessment of respiratory-disease progression and development of new therapies. Small animal ^{3}He lung MRI requires high-spatial-resolution imaging (<500 μm) to obtain acceptable images for visualization of all branches of lung microstructure from the mouse trachea to lung parenchyma. The use of conventional fast-gradient-recalled echo (FGRE) pulse sequences for high-spatial-resolution mouse lung imaging is challenging due to the signal loss caused by significant diffusion-weighting by the imaging gradients, particularly in larger airways where ^{3}He diffusion is maximized. In this chapter, a modified FGRE approach called X-Centric is described for acquiring ^{3}He mouse lung MRI. X-Centric is a center-out technique, allowing high-spatial-resolution, and high signal-to-noise ratio density-weighted imaging, as it is a short-TE method minimizing diffusion decay. Here, we also take advantage of a high-performance insertable-gradient-set interfaced with a clinical MRI system and a custom-built constant-volume ventilator to get the maximum benefits of X-Centric. High-spatial-resolution ^{3}He X-Centric imaging was performed in a phantom and mouse lungs, yielding a nominal resolution of 39 μm and 78 μm respectively. We also demonstrate the feasibility of ^{129}Xe/^{19}F X-Centric MRI in a phantom and in rat lungs.

Keywords: X-Centric, ^{3}He, ^{129}X, ^{19}F mouse, rat, lung, short-TE, x-nuclei, pre-clinical, hyperpolarized, MRI, COPD, CF, BPD, alpha-1 antitrypsin deficiency

1. Introduction

Inhaled hyperpolarized gas lung MRI [1] was proven to be useful for the observation and treatment planning of several pulmonary diseases including chronic obstructive pulmonary disease (COPD) [2–6], asthma, [7–11] and lung cancer [12]. With the combined economic burden of COPD and asthma in Canada, Ontario being $5.7 billion (2011) [13], and lung cancer being the leading cause of cancer deaths worldwide, [14] there has been a growing interest in developing new lung imaging techniques such as hyperpolarized ^{3}He and ^{129}Xe MRI as well as hyperpolarized propane (^{1}H) MRI [15, 16] and thermally polarized inert fluorinated gas (^{19}F) MRI [17–19] to better understand various lung diseases.

Our main focus will be on ^{3}He gas MRI of small animal models of lung disease [20, 21], as it is a promising tool to quantify airway and ventilation abnormalities associated with bronchoconstriction, airway narrowing, and subsequent bronchodilation [22, 23]. Small animal ^{3}He lung MRI normally assumes high spatial

IntechOpen

resolution imaging (<500 μm [22]) in order to obtain acceptable images for the quantitative analysis and visualization of rodent airways and lung parenchyma. However, high-resolution hyperpolarized gas MR imaging has a number of signal-to-noise ratio (SNR) limitations due to the non-renewable nature of the non-equilibrium magnetization, requiring a minimized number of small flip angle radio-frequency (RF) pulses and quite short image acquisition times during a breath-hold which should be as short as a second in duration for the case of mouse lung imaging. Coupled with the issues of high-resolution imaging are the effects of fast diffusion of ^{3}He (~2 cm^2/s) through strong spatial encoding gradients, which can completely destroy the MRI signal in the airways and significantly attenuate the signal in the lung parenchyma [24–26]. There is a need for an imaging method which incorporates specific hardware and novel rapid image acquisition approaches that minimize the signal loss due to all of these mitigating factors and permit fast and high spatial resolution ^{3}He MR imaging of small animal airways and lung microstructure [27]. Such imaging modalities can be used for observation of ventilation heterogeneity, such as in an ovalbumin asthmatic mouse model [22, 27], as well as for pediatric lung applications [28] often requiring much smaller field-of-view (FOV).

The projection-reconstruction (PR) approach is the well-known [29] acquisition method that minimizes ^{3}He diffusion-induced signal decay, as it acquires the k-space center immediately following the excitation pulse and before the imaging gradient starts which avoids significant signal loss occurs [27]. Both PR and spiral/cones acquisitions belong to free induction decay based or apparent transverse relaxation time (T_2*) based methods, acquiring k-space in a non-Cartesian fashion. It has been demonstrated that those methods reduce diffusion-weighting for ^{3}He MRI of rodent lungs [22, 30–34]. In addition, they ensure very short echo-times ((TE) < 200 μs) which minimizes T_2*-weighting, leading to pure gas density weighting [35]. Unfortunately, PR uses a significant number of RF pulses (50,640 views for a 128 × 128 × 128 matrix size and 204,196 for a 256 × 256 × 256 matrix size [36]) or radial projections to sufficiently sample k-space and this naturally leads to reduction of the available SNR from the non-renewable hyperpolarized state [27]. Cones [34] and spiral [28] k-space trajectories normally do not require a significant number of RF tipping or interleaves to fill k-space, but this should still be compensated by using an elongated readout-window which can be difficult to achieve due to the short T_2* of ^{3}He gas in small animal lungs (T_2* < 3 ms, at high field [37]). Commonly, non-Cartesian acquisitions require dedicated k-space interpolating and regridding as well as density-weighting procedures for image reconstruction [27], which often can have smoothing effects and resolution implications. Furthermore, non-Cartesian traversal of k-space by either PR or spiral/cones often requires significant oversampling, which leads to commensurate increases in acquisition time and consequently prohibiting single breath-hold imaging in rodents. Driehuys et al. [22] suggests that ^{3}He MRI measurements of rapid dynamic changes in mouse lungs followed by methacholine challenge can be done more time and cost efficiently with fast 2D Cartesian imaging compared to 3D PR.

An alternative to PR (which may suffer from poor edge resolution and sampling/reconstruction artifacts [18]) for high spatial resolution single-breath 2D imaging of small animal lung employs two separate excitations with inverted read-out gradients to acquire both halves of Cartesian k-space in a center-out fashion to minimize both diffusion-weighting [38, 39] and T_2*-weighting [17]. This technique is known as the X-Centric method [27, 39]. It uses a well-known Fast Gradient-Recalled Echo (FGRE) sequence as its basis [27, 39], so the method can be relatively easy implemented on any clinical MRI scanners [17, 27]. Also, because X-Centric is a Cartesian method, it does not require interpolating, regridding and density-weighting procedures for image reconstruction [17, 27, 39]. It minimizes both gradient-induced diffusion attenuation [27, 39] and T_2*-based signal attenuation [17] at the center of k-space, and does not depend on the image resolution for a chosen FOV and bandwidth (BW_{read}).

In this chapter we present an X-Centric approach developed for a single breath-hold high spatial resolution ^{3}He MRI of mouse lungs. The method takes advantage of a high performance insertable gradient set interfaced with a clinical MRI system and precise custom built constant-volume ventilator. The X-Centric approach is compared to partial-echo FGRE [25] on the basis of SNR efficiency over a range of spatial resolutions in a phantom [27]. The robustness of the X-Centric technique for ^{3}He in-vivo lung imaging of mice is demonstrated [27]. The feasibility of the X-Centric approach to image dissolved hyperpolarized ^{129}Xe in a phantom and with ^{19}F gas in a rat lung [17] is also demonstrated in this chapter.

2. Theoretical background

2.1 ^{3}He MRI

Table 1 summarizes the physical properties of the ^{3}He isotope along with other gases used for inhaled lung MRI [40] such as ^{129}Xe [1, 41], inert fluorinated gases possessing ^{19}F spins [17–19] and propane [16] which is proton-based (^{1}H). It is well-known, that helium gas has the highest self-diffusion coefficient (*D*), which is around 2 cm^2/s for pure helium, and it is around 0.9 cm^2/s, when helium diffuses in air or is part of a helium/air mixture. Its very high diffusivity suggests that high-resolution ^{3}He MRI can be quite challenging due to the induced decay of the MR signal by the applied imaging gradients [22, 24]. However, signal attenuation due to diffusion is not the only reason making high-resolution ^{3}He MRI problematic. In most cases it requires very careful consideration of all MRI related physical properties of ^{3}He and sequence parameter effects, such as the contribution of relaxation times to both signal decay and image blurring [42]. In addition to these

Parameter	C_3H_8 (^{1}H)	SF_6 (^{19}F)	^{3}He	^{129}Xe
Nuclear spin, I	1/2	1/2	1/2	1/2
Gyromagnetic ratio, (MHz rad/T)	267.5	251.6	203.7	74.5
Natural abundance (%)	100	95	1.4×10^{-4}	26
Apparent transverse relaxation time, T_2* (ms)	>1.0	$0.5^a/2.0^b$	$1.5^a/3.2^b$	$2.8^a/2.9^c$
Longitudinal relaxation time, T_1 (s)	5.0	30	90^d	25^d
Self-diffusion coef., D_0 (cm^2/s)	10^{-3}	0.033	2.05	0.061
Diffusion coef. in air, D (cm^2/s)	0.098	0.094	0.86	0.14
b-Values, (s/cm^2)	12	12	1.6	9
Chemical shift range, Δδ (ppm)	20	150	0.8	220
Ostwald solubility $\times 10^{-4}$, L	61	54	850	1700
Cost, per liter	$20	$20	$800	$20/200^e

SF_6 and ^{3}He T_2 values shown within major airway^a and parenchema^b of the rodent lung. ^{129}Xe T_2* values shown for xenon gas^a within the major airway and xenon dissolved^c within lung tissue (barrier) and red blood cells. ^{129}Xe and ^{3}He T_1 values^d measured in rodent lungs after several wash-out (anoxic) breaths of the hyperpolarized gas. Cost of the 86% enriched ^{129}Xe^e.*

Table 1.
Comparison of ^{3}He, ^{129}Xe, inert fluorinated gas and propane.

considerations, one needs to consider the use of special MRI hardware such as a high-performance high-slew-rate imaging gradient set [43] and a very high precision ventilator [27] for in-vivo high-resolution imaging. The high diffusivity of ^{3}He as well as its short relaxation times and MRI hardware limitations should all be taken into account for the proper choice of the pulse sequence when high spatial resolution ^{3}He MRI is the goal.

2.2 Relaxation times

Generally, both longitudinal and apparent transverse relaxation [44] times (T_1 and T_2*) of ^{3}He are not physical constants and they both depend on the main magnetic field strength, its gradients, presence of paramagnetic impurities interacting with the hyperpolarized gas (e.g., oxygen), and finally, diffusivity. Normally, the main mechanism for T_1 decay of hyperpolarized gases (i.e., polarization losses in contrast to conventional thermally polarized spins) is the presence of oxygen in lung [45]. The T_1 decay rate is inversely proportional to the partial oxygen pressure (pO_2) [46]:

$$\frac{1}{T_1} = \frac{1}{T_{1,0}} + \kappa \int_0^{time} pO_2(t)dt \qquad (1)$$

where $T_{1,0}$ is the longitudinal relaxation time expected in the absence of O_2 and κ is the relaxivity of ^{3}He due to the presence of O_2 (0.38 $atm^{-1}\ s^{-1}$ at body temperature [46]).

This suggests that a small number of anoxic pre-breaths or wash-out breaths prior the actual ^{3}He MRI measurements can be helpful for minimizing the oxygen concentration in lung prior to acquisition and administration of hyperpolarized gas. **Table 1** suggests that the T_1 in small animal lungs after applying a number of wash-out breaths can be sufficiently long [47] compared to the typical image acquisition times of 1 s [27] for mice and 10 s for rats [37]. As previous work shows, eight wash-out breaths drastically reduce the O_2 concentration [17, 23, 48]. The value of T_2* for ^{3}He normally varies between the major airways (1.5 $\pm$ 0.25 ms [37]) and lung parenchyma (3.0 $\pm$ 1.0 ms [37]) due to the differences in airway size which have a significant effect on the mode of diffusion (e.g., free diffusion vs. restricted) and amount of signal loss due to diffusion. **Table 1** shows T_2* values obtained for hyperpolarized gas within rat lungs at 3 Tesla. As expected T_2* estimates obtained for the major airways were smaller than the estimates observed in lung parenchyma.

2.3 Signal to noise ratio

An imaging sequence should be optimized to simultaneously ensure maximum SNR and minimal blurring in order to successfully perform high-resolution hyperpolarized ^{3}He MR measurements. Understanding of the mechanisms that affect SNR and contribute to image blurring is the basis for the developing an imaging technique appropriate for hyperpolarized gas imaging. Generally, an expression for the SNR of a FGRE sequence can be expressed as [42]:

$$SNR \propto \Delta x \Delta y \Delta z \sqrt{\frac{N_x N_y N_z}{BW_{read}}} f\left(\rho,\ P, \alpha,\ T_2^*,\ T_1,\ b,\ D\right) \qquad (2)$$

where $\Delta x \Delta y \Delta z$ is the voxel size, $N_x N_y N_z$ is the number of k-space samples in each direction, BW_{read} readout bandwidth and $f(\rho, \ P, \alpha, \ T_2^*, \ T_1, \ b, \ D)$ is the pulse-sequence-dependent function that determines the signal amplitudes at readout for the center of k-space [49]:

$$f(\rho, \ P, \ T_1, \ T_2^* \ \alpha, \ b, \ D) \approx \rho P \sin(\alpha) \exp^{(-TE/T_2^*)} \exp^{(-TR/T_1)} \exp^{(-b \ D)} \quad (3)$$

As it can be seen, the signal amplitudes at readout depend on the density (ρ) and polarization (P) of ^{3}He, flip angle (α), TE, repetition time (TR) and finally, diffusion attenuation [50] introduced by slice select and/or frequency encoding gradients. In order to simultaneously minimize T_1 decay and T_2*-induced blurring and maximize signal, one should use a short-TE (TE < 1 ms) center-out k-space traversal pulse sequence to ensure only density-weighting at the center of k-space. For the case of TE < T_2*, and if the total acquisition time (1–10 s) is much less than T_1 (25–90 s) the pulse sequence dependent function can be expressed as:

$$f(\rho, \ P, \ \alpha, \ b, \ D) \approx \rho P \sin(\alpha) \exp^{(-b \ D)} \quad (4)$$

where b is the b-value, the diffusion weighting factor that depends on the diffusion gradient duration and magnitude (which in this case are imaging gradients); and D is the diffusion coefficient of ^{3}He in the lung (0.1–2 cm^2/s) [37, 50].

2.4 Flip angle

Let us consider each factor in Eq. (4) individually in order to optimize this function. As the hyperpolarized magnetization is not renewable due to the its non-equilibrium nature, it needs to be spent (flipped by RF pulses) very efficiently. A single 90° RF pulse can effectively waste all of the available magnetization. We start with the two approaches of setting flip angles in hyperpolarized gas MRI. The first method is the Constant Flip Angle (CFA) approach [51] or small flip angle approach (1° < flip angle <10°). Using a CFA approach, the optimal flip angle (α_{opt}), which provides the highest signal for sequential phase encode ordering, is expressed as [51]:

$$\alpha_{opt} = \tan^{-1}\sqrt{2/(N_y N_z)} \quad (5)$$

Unfortunately, the use of the optimal flip angle given by Eq. (5) leads to significant signal decay due to the constant-value RF pulses applied during k-space acquisition. As an example, for a 2D case where N_y = 128 and α_{opt} = 7.1° the signal decays by ~60% across the k-space). An undesirable consequence of such decay is reduced image resolution as result of the RF pulse "history" during k-space acquisition. Point-spread-function (PSF) simulations for a 2D case with center-out phase encode ordering (**Figure 1**) confirmed that the CFA approach leads to image blurring (Full Width at Half Maximum (FWHM) = 1.5 pixels) [47]. This signal decay-induced image blurring can be eliminated by using a Variable Flip Angle (VFA) approach (1° < flip angle <90°) [52]. VFA mitigates signal loss during image acquisition (i.e., blurring) by ensuring a constant signal for each phase-encode line by starting with a low flip angle and incrementing the flip angle of each RF pulse, line after line [52]. The flip angle for each ith phase-encode line of a VFA sequence can be calculated from the following equation [47]:

$$\alpha_i = \tan^{-1}\left[\frac{\exp\left(-(N_yN_z - i)TR/T_1\right)}{\sqrt{N_yN_z - i}}\right] \tag{6}$$

For the case where the total image acquisition time is much less than T_1 (T_1 typically >10 sec under normal conditions), Eq. (6) takes the simpler form [47]:

$$\alpha_i \approx \tan^{-1}\left[\frac{1}{\sqrt{N_yN_z - i}}\right] \tag{7}$$

For a 2D case (N_y = 128), α_1 = 5.1° and α_{128} = 90°, producing no CFA-like signal decay, and consequently, no image blurring due to RF pulse "history" [47]. Simulations have shown that VFA only shows blurring of 1.2 pixels due to discrete sampling [47] and because of these benefits this method is preferable for high spatial resolution ^{3}He imaging.

2.5 *b*-Value

Eq. (4) suggests that signal decay due to diffusion is the main reason the MR signal degradation (assuming minimal T_1 and T_2^* induced blurring and signal loss) and consequently poses as the main difficulty for high spatial resolution ^{3}He imaging. **Figure 2** shows the calculated NMR signal as a function of *b*-value for two different diffusion coefficients, typical for a small animal airways and lung parenchyma respectively [37]. It can be seen that for a *b*-value >3.5 s/cm^2, the signal intensity in the airway is almost zero and there is a 60% loss of signal for lung parenchyma. Let us consider the dependence of *b*-value on the diffusion gradient duration and magnitude. In general, the *b*-value for any gradient waveforms can be calculated from the first principles [42]:

$$b = \gamma^2 \int_0^{t_1} \left[\int_0^{t} G(t')\, dt' \right]^2 dt \tag{8}$$

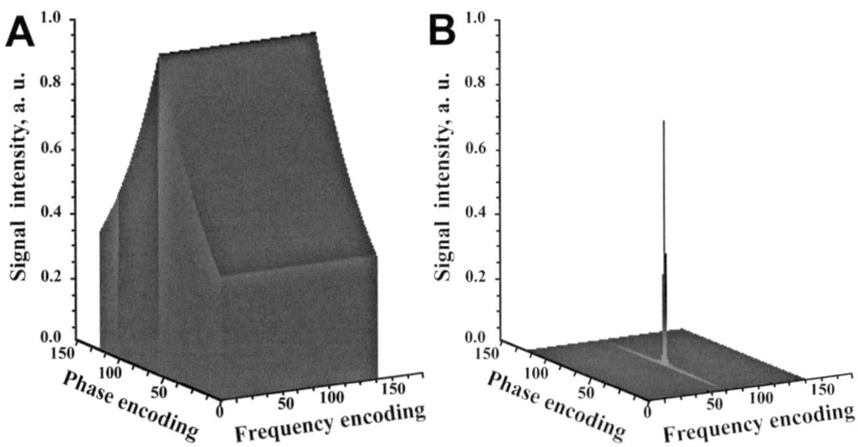

Figure 1.
Point spread function simulation for the CFA approach (a) the k-space is simulated for hyperpolarized CFA ^{3}He signal of a 128 × 128 pixel object with α_{opt} = 7.12° (Eq. (5)) and infinite T_1. (b) Fourier transform of (a) revealing the PSF [47]. The calculated FWHM of the PSF indicates significant blurring (1.5 pixels) in the phase-encode direction [47]. The observed blurring is due to both RF pulse history of non-recoverable magnetization and discrete sampling [47]. Variable flip angle only shows blurring of 1.2 pixels due to discrete sampling [47]. Figure adapted from Ouriadov et al. [47].

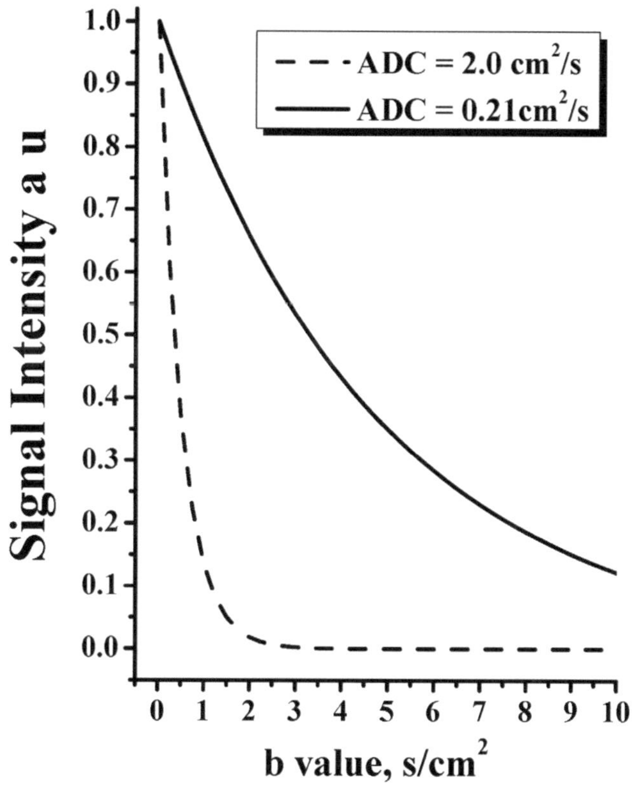

Figure 2.
Dependence of NMR signal on b*-value for two different diffusion coefficients of ³He calculated from the diffusion term of Eq. (4). The dashed line curve represents signal obtained for a* D *value that is typical for airways (free diffusion) and the solid line curve represents signal obtained for a typical* D *value in lung parenchyma. Plot shows that for a* b*-value >3.5 s/cm², the signal intensity in the airway is almost zero and there is 60% of signal loss for lung parenchyma.*

where γ is gyromagnetic ratio, G is gradient amplitude and t, t_1 is gradient duration. Unfortunately, Eq. (8) cannot be analytically simplified further for a gradient waveform specific to the frequency encoding imaging gradient. For a relatively simple diffusion gradient waveform such as two bipolar rectangular pulses, the b-value can be calculated based on the following equation [53]:

$$b = -\frac{2}{3}\gamma^2 G^2 \delta^2 t_d \text{ with } t_d = \left[\Delta - \frac{\delta}{3}\right], \qquad (9)$$

where δ is the diffusion gradient duration, Δ is a distance between two gradient pulses and t_d is the diffusion observation time. Note, that b-value strongly depends on the gradient duration ($\delta^2 t_d$ = time^3) then the magnitude (G^2), which suggests that minimizing the gradient duration reduces the b-value and consequently minimizes the signal loss. This is especially critical for high-resolution ^{3}He imaging, as the imaging gradient magnitude cannot be really decreased when trying to achieve high spatial resolution, or small FOV for mice.

2.6 X-centric

As ^{3}He gas has the highest self-diffusion coefficient of the usable hyperpolarized gases and it is a physical constant, the diffusion weighting b-value due to the application of frequency encoding gradient or x-gradient should be minimized as much as possible. A full-echo FGRE pulse sequence ensures the highest *b*-value (and subsequent signal loss) for gradient echo based sequences [22, 25]. The use of a partial-echo (partial in the x-gradient direction, 62.5% sampled points) FGRE pulse sequence can significantly reduce the *b*-value compared to the full echo FGRE due to reduction in readout time; however, even this reduced *b*-value can be still large enough (>2.0 s/cm^2) to completely destroy MR signal in some lung geometries such as in the case of high spatial resolution ^{3}He imaging in small animals [22, 27]. The main limitation of FGRE is the undesirable dependence of the *b*-value on the x-gradient making this sequence not very suitable for high-resolution ^{3}He imaging. However, it is possible to modify the original FGRE sequence, so it ensures minimal *b*-values due to x-gradients and full independence of the *b*-value from the image resolution for the chosen field-of-view (FOV) and BW_{read}. A modified or X-Centric FGRE pulse sequence is presented in **Figure 3**. The idea of the X-Centric FGRE pulse sequence is straightforward. It acquires half of an echo in the x-direction by starting at the center of k-space then repeats the same k-space line but with the x-gradient inverted in order to collect the second half of the echo in x-direction. **Figure 4** shows part of an experimental x-gradient waveform (nominal resolution 78 μm) from the start of the line acquisition until the center of the k_x line for partial-echo (open squares and dashed line) and X-Centric (solid squares and solid line) FGRE pulse sequences. The area of the pre-phasing gradient shown on the plot is equal to area of the main readout gradient lobe for both acquisition methods. **Figure 4** suggests that the X-Centric FGRE should decrease *b*-value at $k_x = 0$ due to the much shorter diffusion time and smaller pre-phasing gradient magnitude leading to higher signal at the center of k-space.

The X-Centric approach requires two discrete acquisitions for each k-space line making the method twice as long in acquisition time compared to a conventional partial-echo FGRE approach for a chosen spatial resolution and matrix size [17, 27, 39]. Though, this is not a significant cost to achieve high-resolution imaging of the lungs of small animals, the scan time can be further reduced by using a partial-echo method in the phase-encoding direction [17, 27, 39]. Note, that the use of a partial-echo method in the phase-encoding direction makes the X-Centric scan time only 10% longer than the partial-echo FGRE sequence for a similar spatial resolution and matrix size [27].

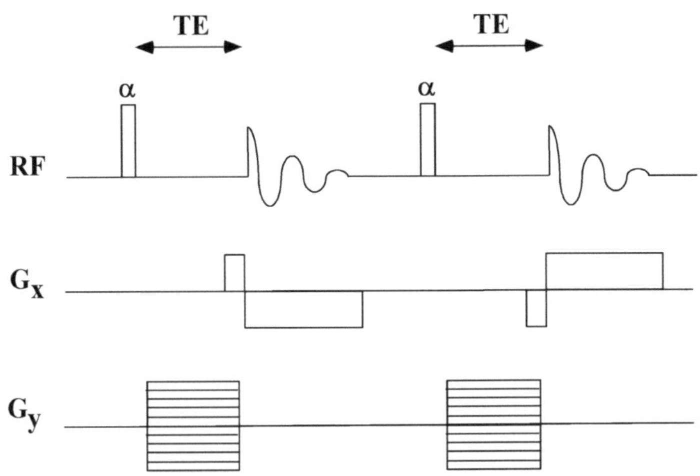

Figure 3.
Pulse sequence timing diagram of X-centric acquisition scheme. The X-centric approach minimizes signal loss due to diffusion since the number of k-space points acquired before the center of the k_x line is significantly reduced. Figure adapted from Ouriadov et al. [27].

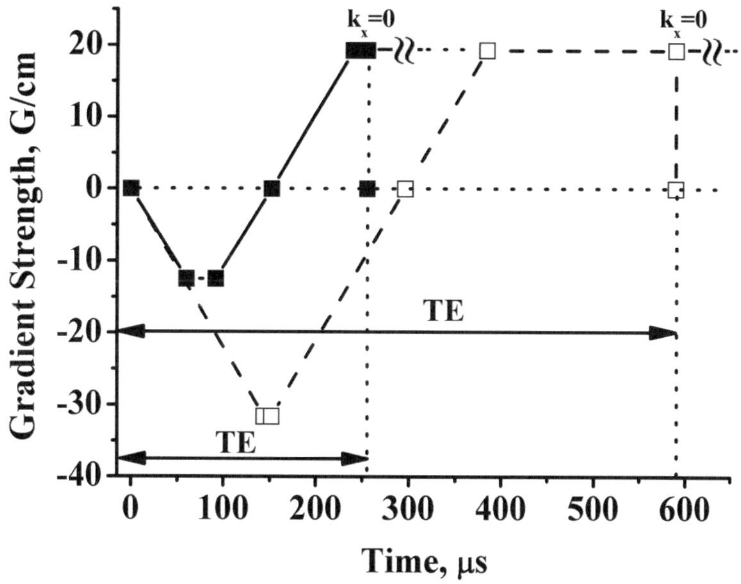

Figure 4.
Expanded view of the readout gradient waveform in partial-echo FGRE (open squares and dashed line) and X-centric (solid squares and solid line) for acquisitions with 256 × 256 image matrix FOV = 2 × 2 cm², and BW_{read} = 62.5 kHz [27]. X-centric waveform has a shorter TE (mainly determined by the duration of the phase-encoding gradient) and much smaller area compared to the partial-echo FGRE waveform resulting in a decreased b-value at k_x = 0 [27]. Both X-centric and FGRE gradient waveforms show the readout gradient until k_x = 0 *point only [27]. Figure adapted from Ouriadov et al. [27].*

2.7 Diffusion attenuation

The exact *b*-value for gradient waveforms presented in **Figure 4** can be calculated from Eq. (8). Thus, *b*-values calculated for the partial-echo and X-Centric FGRE (256 × 256 matrix size) were 2.29 and 0.061 s/cm^2 respectively. **Figure 2** indicates that a *b*-value more than 2.0 s/cm^2 leads to the complete signal decay in the major airway which is a significant limitation for high spatial resolution ^{3}He imaging of the mouse lung. In contrast, the X-Centric sequence should theoretically ensure minimal signal decay for given diffusion coefficients. Note that for the unrestricted ^{3}He diffusion case the theoretical SNR (SNR_{theor}) should depend only on *b*-value and *D*:

$$SNR_{theor} = S_0 \exp^{(-bD)} \quad (10)$$

where S_0 is the initial signal (S_0 = 1), *D* is the free ^{3}He self-diffusion coefficient (2.0 cm^2/s) and *b* takes on a value determined by the chosen FOV and BW_{read}.

According to Eq. (2), for the case of the high-resolution 2D ^{3}He phantom imaging, the SNR should generally depend on the diffusion attention, image resolution, BW_{read} and the first flip angle in the VFA scheme [27]:

$$SNR \propto P\rho \sin(\alpha_1)\ \Delta x \Delta y \sqrt{\frac{N_x N_y}{BW_{read}}} \exp^{(-bD)} \quad (11)$$

as Δx, Δy can be expressed through FOVs and N_x, and N_y Eq. (11) can be rewritten as

$$SNR \propto P\rho \sin(\alpha_1) \; \frac{FOV_x FOV_y}{N_x N_y} \sqrt{\frac{N_x N_y}{BW_{read}}} \exp^{(-bD)} \tag{12}$$

If one keeps FOV, BW_{read}, ^3He polarization and volume constant across all phantom measurements, then the SNR comparison between the partial-echo and X-Centric FGRE can be done by normalizing the experimental SNR by the first flip angle in the VFA scheme (α_1) and matrix size ($\sqrt{N_x N_y}$). Thus, for a SNR normalized by the respective first applied flip angle and matrix size, one can write the following expression [27]:

$$SNR_{nor} = \frac{SNR}{\sin(\alpha_1)} \sqrt{N_x N_y} = Const \cdot \exp^{(-bD)} \tag{13}$$

where $Const = P\rho \; \frac{FOV_x FOV_y}{\sqrt{BW_{read}}}$. This final SNR_{nor} equation can be used for SNR comparisons of the phantom images obtained for different resolutions with the partial-echo and X-Centric FGRE methods; also this equation is similar to Eq. (10).

2.8 Phantom imaging

A plastic 10 mL syringe filled with hyperpolarized ^3He was used to validate the X-Centric sequence for high spatial resolution imaging [27]. **Figure 5** shows a 2D coronal view whole projection phantom images obtained for partial-echo (top panel) and X-Centric (bottom panel) FGRE for five different resolutions. Images start from 64 × 64 matrix size and end with 512 × 512 from left to the right [27]. The images indicate that at low nominal resolution (625 μm, 64 × 64 matrix size) there is no qualitative or visual difference in the SNR between the images obtained for the partial-echo and X-Centric FGRE. However, there is virtually no signal in phantom images obtained with partial-echo FGRE when nominal resolution is

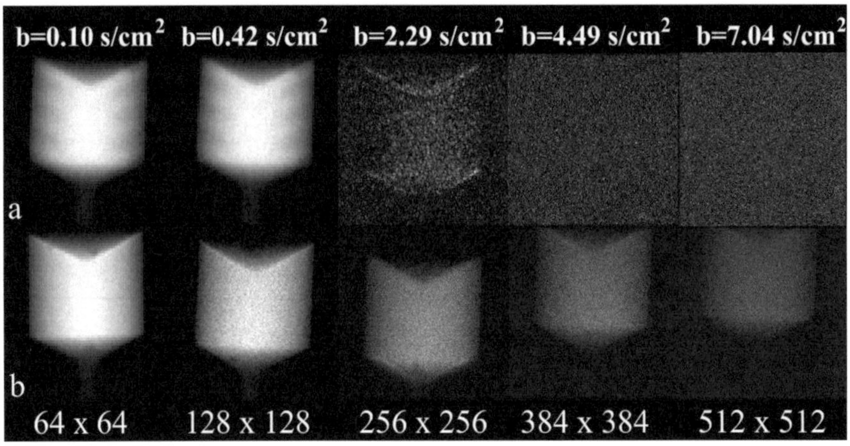

Figure 5.
Hyperpolarized ^3He phantom images (64 × 64, 128 × 128, 256 × 256, 384 × 384, 512 × 512 from left to right with a FOV = 2 × 2 cm², and BW_{read} = 62.5 kHz) obtained in the coronal plane at 1 atm gas pressure (D = 2.0 cm²/s) for image acquisition times up to 6.7 s for: (a) partial-echo FGRE (top row with b-values ranging from 0.1 to 7.04 s/cm² at k_x = 0) and (b) X-centric (bottom row with a b-value equal to 0.061 s/cm² at k_x = 0) [27]. Whereas the X-centric images demonstrate only a gradual loss in signal intensity with increasing image matrix, the partial-echo FGRE had no signal intensity for images with matrix sizes of 384 × 384 and 512 × 512. The partial-echo FGRE image obtained for 256 × 256 has been filtered with a Hanning filter to increase signal intensity. The changes of syringe vertical position are due to the slight displacement of the syringe inside the holder between fresh gas administrations. Figure adapted from Ouriadov et al. [27].

greater than 256 × 256 (78 μm nominal resolution). As expected, the signal intensity of the images obtained with X-Centric gradually decays with increasing nominal resolution and decreasing flip angle (because the first pulse for VFA is a function of resolution, Eq. (7)) but even for 512 × 512 matrix size (39 μm nominal resolution) it does not go below the noise floor as is seen in the case of the partial-echo FGRE. The SNR_{nor} dependence on resolution (bottom axis) and/or b-value (top axis, partial-echo case only) for the phantom images obtained with the partial-echo (solid squares and solid line) and X-Centric FGRE (solid circles and solid line) is plotted in **Figure 6**. Clearly, the SNR_{nor} obtained for the X-Centric did not depend on image resolution, i.e., diffusion attenuation was minimal even for very high image resolution (39 μm). The experimental phantom results were consistent with the predicted SNR (SNR_{theor}) calculated based on Eq. (10) for the partial-echo (open squares and dashed line) and X-Centric FGRE (open circles and dashed line). Eqs. (10) and (13) indicate that for the case of unrestricted ^{3}He diffusion (D = 2 cm^2/s) one should observe minor signal loss (~10%) using X-Centric and almost 100% signal loss using the partial-echo FGRE for a nominal resolution greater than 78 μm. Thus our consideration of the factors determining the SNR for high spatial resolution ^{3}He MR measurements shows that in the case of relatively short TR and TE (pulse sequence parameters for 256 × 256 matrix size are present in **Table 2**) diffusion is the major reason for signal loss. Using the X-Centric method, diffusion decay due to the x-gradients is significantly minimized. It should be noted that we observed a slight

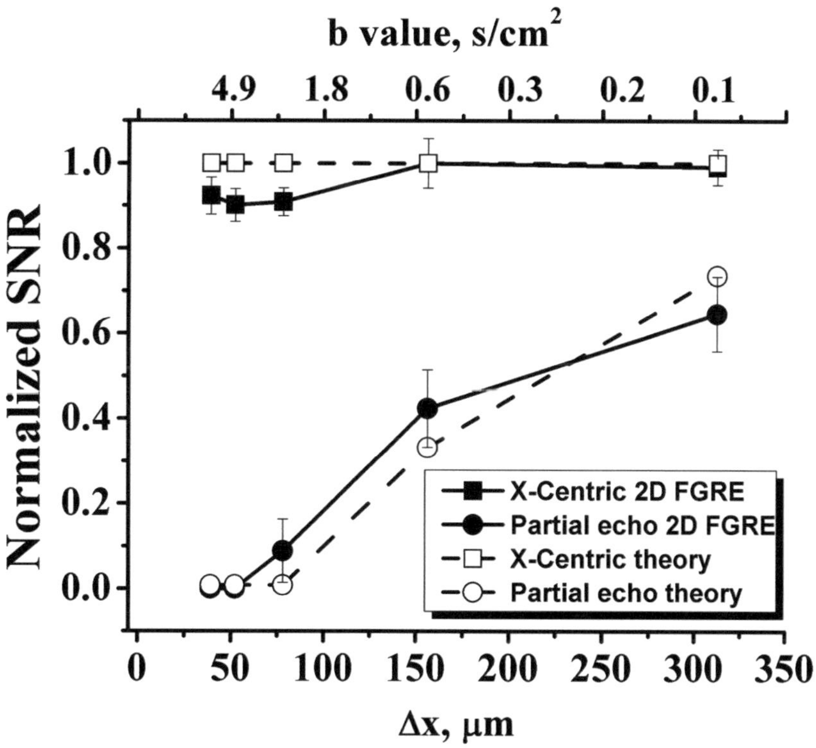

Figure 6.
Scaled normalized SNR of the phantom images (Eq. (13)) shown in Figure 5a and b versus spatial resolution (bottom horizontal axes) and b-value (top horizontal axes) for: (i) partial-echo FGRE (solid circles and solid line) and X-centric (solid squares and solid line) acquisitions [27]. These data are consistent with the predicted data (open squares and dashed line for partial-echo and open circles and dashed line for X-centric) based on the calculated b-values (Eq. (13)) [27]. This plot shows independence of normalized SNR from image resolution for the x-centric acquisition schemes [27]. The b-value axis (calculated for experimental x-gradient waveform based on Eq. (8)) applies only to the partial-echo FGRE curves as the b-values for X-centric curves were constant (0.061 s/cm^2) as a function of resolution [27]. Figure adapted from Ouriadov et al. [27].

	^{3}He MRI	^{129}Xe MRI	^{19}F MRI
TE/TR (ms)	0.70/3.7	0.81/50.0	.50/4.0
Flip angle	3.2° (VFA)	6.4° (CFA)	70 ° (EA)
FOV (mm^2)	20 × 20	250 × 250	60 × 60
Matrix size	256 × 160	128 × 80	64 × 40
Number of averages	1	1	60
Slice orientation	Axial/coronal	Axial/coronal	Axial/coronal
Pixel size (mm^3)	0.078 × 0.078	1.9 × 1.9 × 300	0.94 × 0.84
Scan time (s)	1.1	>8	>10
MRI scanner	GE 3 T MR750	Philip. 3 T Achieva	Philip. 3 T Achieva

VFA = variable flip angle; CFA = constant flipped angle; EA = Ernst angle; FOV = field of view; TR = relaxation time; TE = echo-time.

Table 2.
MRI acquisition parameters for methods in this chapter.

decrease of the SNR_{nor} (around 10%) for a nominal resolutions better than 75 μm (**Figure 6**) which were likely due to T_2* decay because as resolution increases, TE becomes longer due to the longer duration of phase-encoding gradient. Nevertheless, X-Centric phantom images show no evidence of image blurring due to the RF pulse history or T_2*-based signal decay in the frequency/phase encoding directions. The phantom measurements have confirmed that significant diffusion attenuation induced by the x-gradient with the partial-echo FGRE sequence can be the main restriction for high spatial resolution ^{3}He imaging of the lung.

3. High spatial resolution imaging of mouse lung

3.1 Animal preparation

The animal protocol was approved by the Animal Use Subcommittee of the University Council on Animal Care at the University of Western Ontario, London, Ontario, Canada and the Animal Care Committee at Merck Frosst Canada, Kirkland, Quebec, Canada. Each mouse (BALB/c) was pretreated with Midazolam (1 mg/kg) intraperitoneally (i.p.) 5 min before anesthesia with ketamine (95 mg/kg, i.p.) and xylazine (6.4 mg/kg, i.p.). Following anesthesia, the tail vein was cannulated (26 GA Abbott catheter) to maintain anesthesia with ketamine (30 mg/kg) and xylazine (2 mg/kg) every 40 min. To allow artificial mechanical ventilation, the trachea was cannulated by tracheotomy using an 18 GA Teflon catheter. A line for administration of pancuronium (0.8 mg/kg, i.p.) was established using a 26 GA cannula to allow for injections after the mouse was being ventilated inside the scanner. Other physiological instrumentation included ECG and a rectal temperature probe (SA Instruments Inc., Stony Brook, NY).

3.2 Ventilation

It was a very challenging task to design a ventilator to ventilate mice inside an MRI because of the restrictions due to the high magnetic field environment and the requirement to accurately deliver very small tidal volumes of gas to the lungs of mice at a high ventilation rate. Under spontaneous breathing, the mouse maintains its oxygenation with a tidal volume less than 0.1 ml [54, 55]. Because of the dead space volume within the tubing necessary for connecting mouse airways to the ventilator, the mouse was normally ventilated with tidal volume of 0.2 ml (8 ml/kg). In this range, the amount of the ventilating gas (or fresh gas) getting compressed in the gas line could significantly reduce the portion of fresh gas entering the lungs for gas exchange. Without a proper correction for this effect, adequate ventilation would not be achieved at this ventilating setting. In many cases, the ventilation was set with a much larger tidal volume (>10 ml/kg) at a slower ventilation rate (60–90 bpm). Since lung volume under spontaneous breathing is only 0.3–0.4 ml [56], the larger tidal volume approach could overextend the airways. As a result, many mice were observed to expire shortly after the ventilation, impeding the completion of studies.

To resolve these problems, we modified a flexiVent ventilator (**Figure 7**, Scireq, Montreal, QC, Canada) that incorporated real-time monitoring of volume and pressure to allow corrections of the gas compression effect. To minimize the gas line volume and ensure the effectiveness of ventilation, a non-metal swing valve was designed and placed close to the animal (inside the scanner) to regulate the gas flow. Different than the pneumatic valves normally used in the magnetic environment, the swing valve was connected to two driving solenoid valves (which reside far away from the high magnetic field) via two multiple-section light-weight carbon fiber rods. This mechanical design enabled fast open/close activations. The activation of a solenoid valve pulls the swing valve to close the ports on one side and open the ports on the other side. Two solenoid valves were activated in sequence to generate a swing motion that opens and closes the ports on the respective sides alternately. This swing motion was synchronized with the plunging motion of the piston that drives the gas into the lung to form a ventilation cycle. Because of the fast response of the swing valve, the modified flexiVent ventilator is capable of performing the forced oscillation method to access pulmonary mechanics. To minimize oxygen-induced depolarization (T_1 decay) of hyperpolarized ^{3}He gas, the flexiVent ventilator was modified to deliver breathing gas and hyperpolarized ^{3}He gas separately using two individual syringes. The ventilation system was integrated to the MR scanner (**Figure 7**) using custom-designed LabView software (National Instruments) to allow ventilation-synchronous acquisition. Following the animal preparation, the animal was connected to the ventilator and ventilated using a tidal volume of 8 ml/kg at 100 bpm and was placed inside the scanner. The breath-hold time for imaging was 1 s.

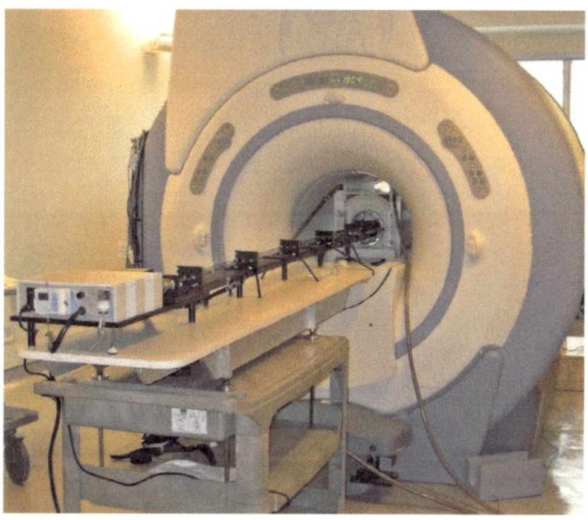

Figure 7.
GE 3 T clinical MRI scanner using an external gradient set for rodents and the integrated custom-built flexiVent ventilator for mice.

3.3 ^{3}He polarization and delivery

^{3}He gas was polarized using an optical pumping spin-exchange system (Helispin™, GE Healthcare, Durham, NC). The ^{3}He gas was typically polarized for at least 8 hours to achieve a polarization over 35%. Prior to transferring the hyperpolarized ^{3}He gas to a 150 mL Tedlar bag (Jensen Inert Products, Coral Springs, FL), the bag was carefully washed with N_2 gas three times to eliminate any oxygen contamination. Following the gas filling, the ^{3}He bag was placed inside a custom-made plexiglass chamber and connected to a ^{3}He intake line of the ventilator. The chamber was then placed within the homogenous B_0 field inside the scanner to conserve ^{3}He polarization (T_1 = ~43 min). To facilitate gas intake by the ventilator, the pressure in the chamber was kept at 3 cm-H_2O during the gas delivery.

To validate the X-Centric imaging method, 2 mL at 1 atm of the hyperpolarized ^{3}He gas was drawn into a 10 mL syringe for phantom testing [27].

3.4 MRI hardware and sequence parameters

Hyperpolarized ^{3}He MR imaging was performed on a GE clinical scanner (3 T, Excite 12.0) which was converted using a home-made insert gradient set (**Figure 8**, maximum gradient at 50 G/cm, 17 cm in diameter, slew rate = 2100 mT/m/s) [43] to allow high spatial resolution imaging for mice. This high performance insert gradient set was used for phantom and mouse imaging [27]. A quadrature birdcage RF coil for mice (**Figure 9**, 3 cm in diameter and 6 cm in length, Morris Instruments, Ottawa, ON) was used for ^{3}He imaging (97.3 MHz) [27]. The coil was driven using a 8 kW AMT 3 T90 RF power amplifier (GE Healthcare, Waukesha, WI)

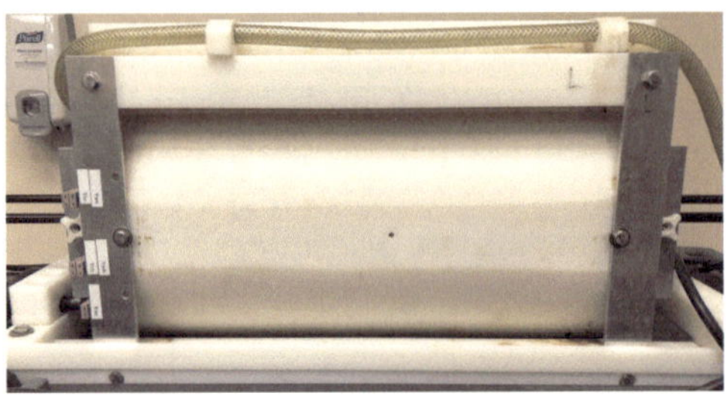

Figure 8.
High performance water cooled insertable gradient set with maximum gradient at 50 G/cm, 17 cm in diameter and slew rate = 2100 mT/m/s used for high-resolution ^{3}He imaging.

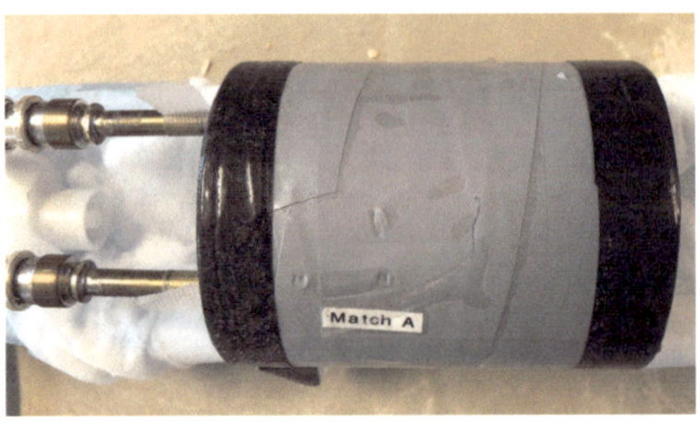

Figure 9.
A quadrature birdcage RF coil for mice (Morris instruments, Ottawa, ON): 97.3 MHz, 3 cm in diameter and 6 cm in length, was used for used for high-resolution ^{3}He imaging.

using a manufacturer-supplied T/R switch and preamplifier tuned to 97.3 MHz. Typical rectangular 90° RF pulse lengths were 100 μs [27]. A VFA RF pulse trajectory was employed to reduce blurring due to RF de-polarization [47, 52]. Center-out sampling in the phase-encoding direction was used [52]. The VFA pulses were calibrated as described in [48].

3.5 Image reconstruction

A custom-made IDL6.4 (ITT Visual Information Solutions, Boulder, CO) routine was used for off-line Fast Fourier transformation (FFT) of the k-space data. For reconstruction of the X-Centric data, a combination of both halves of k-space was applied prior to the inverse Fourier transformation as follows. To form a full line of k-space data in the read-out direction, the two half-echo data sets were combined [17]. Each half-echo data set included two additional points (BW_{read} = 62.5 kHz dwell time was 8 μs) prior to $k_x = 0$ which can be thought of as partial-echo factor of 0.505 for each half.

Acquisition of a few extra k_x data points is helpful since the presence of background gradients can shift the origin of k-space by one or more points resulting in mis-sampling or causing image artifacts [57]. These extra k-space points (only two) were removed before combining the two halves of k-space prior to reconstruction [17]. The disadvantage of this approach is that this leads to a b-value three times larger and longer TR due to the extra sampled points. However, phantom results demonstrate that this increased b-value (b = 0.061 s/cm^2) is still quite practical, ensuring minimal mis-sampling even in the presence of significant background-gradients and gradient-induced eddy currents [17, 27, 39]. Collection of the extra four k_x points (two points per half) for each k_x line results in a 1.5% over-sampling factor for a 256 × 256 matrix size as an example [27].

3.6 In-vivo imaging

X-Centric sequence parameters for the highest image resolution (78 μm) are shown in **Table 2**. *In-vivo* high-resolution 2D whole lung projection ^{3}He mouse lung images obtained for partial-echo (top panels) and X-Centric (bottom panels) FGRE acquisitions for three different matrix sizes are shown in **Figure 10** (axial view) and **Figure 11** (coronal view). Images were obtained during a 1 s breath-hold following three wash-out ^{3}He pre-breaths. It is easy to see that both the axial and coronal images of the mouse lung obtained at high spatial resolution (78 μm) with X-Centric demonstrates visible signal in the major airways. Axial and coronal images of mouse lung obtained for the same resolution setting with partial-echo FGRE show no signal in the trachea as well as lower SNR in the lung periphery. The mean SNR for X-Centric images computed from the mouse lung airways and parenchyma [58] were 25 and 14 respectively [27]. The corresponding mean SNR for the partial-echo FGRE computed for airways and parenchyma were 1.8 (which is less than the Rose criteria of SNR = 5, [59]) and 8 respectively [27]. The large b-value of the partial-echo FGRE led to complete signal destruction in the major airways where ^{3}He experiences near-free diffusion (D = 2 cm^2/s). Besides this, a relatively long TE (1.2 ms [27]) in combination with a shorter T_2* (**Table 1**) in the mouse lung trachea also significantly contributes to signal decay together with diffusion losses. In comparison to the larger airways, the lung parenchyma within the images obtained with partial-echo FGRE still shows some signal, which is not surprising considering that the ^{3}He diffusion was significantly restricted here (D = 0.21 cm^2/s [37]) and T_2* value was long enough (**Table 1**).

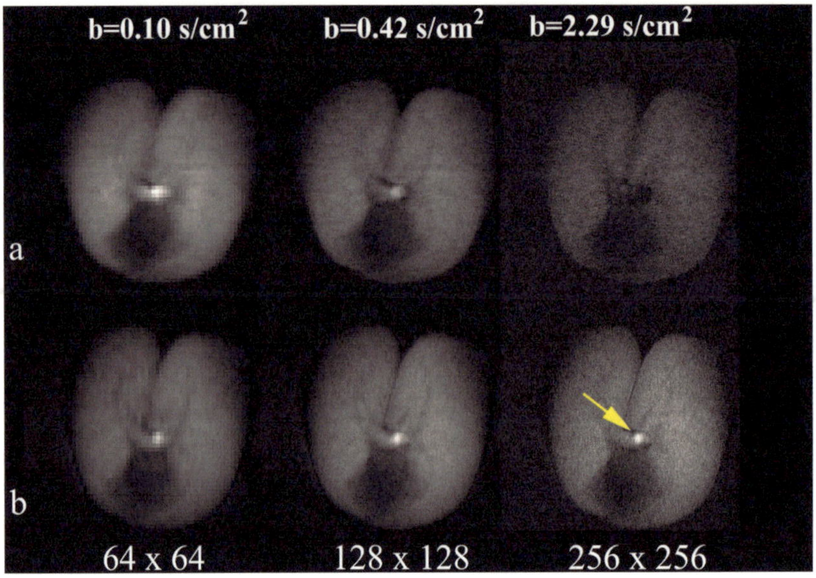

Figure 10.
Hyperpolarized ^{3}He mouse images (64 × 64, 128 × 128, 256 × 256 from left to right FOV = 2 × 2 cm^2, and BW_{read} = 62.5 kHz) obtained in the axial plane using a single breath hold with image acquisition times up to 1.1 s for: partial-echo FGRE (top panel, b-values ranging from 0.1 to 2.29 s/cm^2 at k_x = 0) and X-centric (bottom panel, b-value equals 0.061 s/cm^2 at k_x = 0) [27]. At high-resolution (256 × 256), the partial-echo FGRE images show no signal intensity in the trachea in contrast with the high-resolution X-centric images due to differences in the incidental diffusion weighting in the large airway compared to the lung parenchyma (shown by the arrow) [27]. Figure adapted from Ouriadov et al. [27].

The larger SNR in the major airway (X-Centric mouse lung images) compared to the lung parenchyma is likely due to the higher ^{3}He density in trachea and reasonably short TE used in X-Centric sequence (0.7 ms [27]).

It is useful to calculate the SNR efficiency (ϒ) of the X-Centric and partial-echo FGRE acquisitions was using the following equation [60]:

$$\Upsilon = \frac{SNR/(\Delta x \Delta y)}{\sqrt{T_{scan}}} \tag{14}$$

where T_{scan} is the total imaging time (in s) and SNR was measured based on the mean of Region of Interests (ROI) placed in the rodent lung airways and parenchyma divided by the standard deviation measured in the background (noise) [58]. Thus, X-Centric was 13.4 times more efficient than the partial-echo FGRE sequence for the case of the major airways [27] and 1.7 times more efficient in case of MR imaging of parenchyma [27] (**Figure 11**).

3.7 Limitations

One of the limitations of the X-Centric method is the need to use the FFT for image reconstruction from two half-echo k-space samples rather than a single k-space. Instead, one can use a single half-echo k-space and Partial Fourier Reconstruction (PFR) [61]. To test this idea we used the Projection Onto Convex Sets (POCS) method [62] to reconstruct a phantom image for 130 × 256 (2 + 128 × 256) matrix size (**Figure 5b**). **Figure 12** shows phantom images obtained with PFR (left column) and FFT (right column) for three different matrix sizes. The following SNR values were obtained for the presented images: SNR = 39 (160 × 256, PFR); SNR = 54 (160 × 256, zero-filling in x-direction and then FFT); SNR = 45

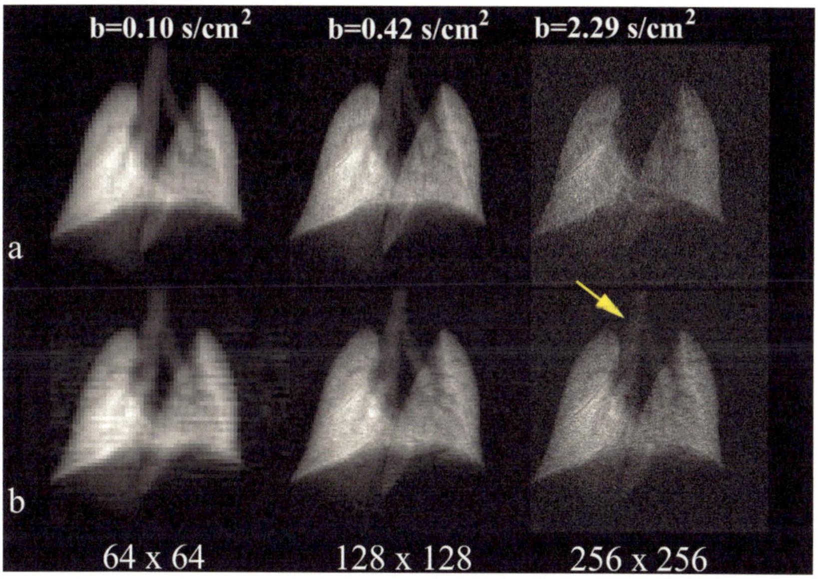

Figure 11.
Hyperpolarized ^{3}He mouse images (64 × 64, 128 × 128, 256 × 256 from left to right FOV = 2 × 2 cm^2, and BW_{read} = 62.5 kHz) obtained in the coronal plane within a single breath hold with image acquisition times up to 1.1 s for: partial-echo FGRE (top panel, b-values ranging from 0.1 to 2.29 s/cm^2 at k_x = 0) and X-centric (bottom panel, b-value equals 0.061 s/cm^2 at k_x = 0) [27]. At high-resolution (256 × 256), the partial-echo FGRE images show no signal intensity in the trachea in contrast with the high-resolution X-centric images due to differences in the incidental diffusion weighting in the large airway compared to the lung parenchyma (shown by the arrow) [27]. Figure adapted from Ouriadov et al. [27].

(130 × 256, PFR); and SNR = 58 (256 × 160, zero-filling in y-direction and then FFT). The results confirm that the FFT with zero-filling approach gives better SNR than the PFR method for 160 × 256 matrix (39 vs. 54). We have calculated the efficiency of half-echo acquisition (130 × 256, SNR = 45) reconstructed with PRF and X-Centric (256 × 160, 62.5% under-sampling in y-direction, SNR = 58) reconstructed with FFT in order to compare imaging methods. Thus, the calculated efficiency ratio is 0.87 (Eq. (14), with T_{scan} = 256 and 160 + 160 y-gradient steps for the half-echo and the X-Centric respectively). This shows that a half-echo acquisition is 13% less efficient than X-Centric, which reflects smaller SNR due to the 50.1% sampling vs. 62.5% sampling for the case of X-Centric, but half-echo acquisition is ~200 ms faster due to the doubling of y-gradient steps for X-Centric. We believe that our half-echo acquisition vs. X-Centric results indicate that the half-echo approach is 20% faster but 10% less SNR efficient than X-Centric.
A structured phantom needs to be used for probing the potential smoothing effects and resolution implications following the Partial Fourier Reconstruction.

3.8 Future role of X-Centric

The focus of this chapter is a presentation of a fast and SNR efficient imaging method for high spatial resolution imaging of mouse lungs that include both the airways and lung parenchyma. Such a technique can be potentially used for mapping the morphological changes and ventilation heterogeneity associated with rodent models of asthma or ovalbumin-challenged model (OVA). **Figure 13** shows an example of ventilation heterogeneity maps obtained for a sham mouse (right column) and OVA treated mouse (left column). The figure compares increased (a and c) and decreased (b and d) ventilation heterogeneity indexes from a sham mouse (left column) and an OVA mouse (right column) under similar increases in

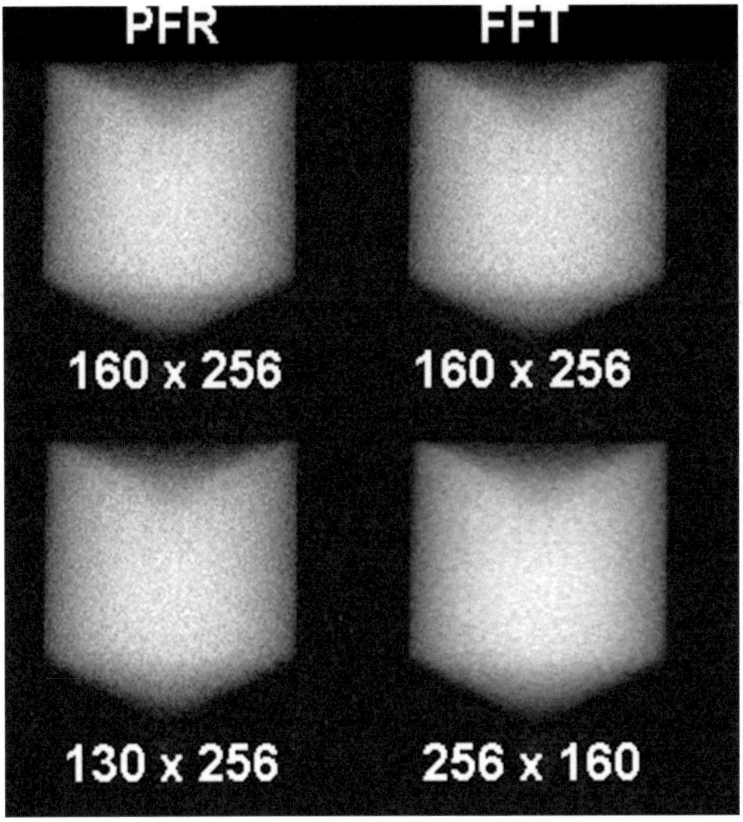

Figure 12.
Phantom images obtained with partial Fourier reconstruction (PFR, left column) and fast Fourier reconstruction (FFT, right column) for three different matrix sizes are shown. The open source partial Fourier reconstruction (projection onto convex sets (POCS), 2013) was obtained from the official MatLab web site. The following signal-to-noise ratio (SNR) values were obtained for the presented images: SNR = 39 (160 × 256, PFR); SNR = 54 (160 × 256, FFT); SNR = 45 (130 × 256, PFR); and SNR = 58 (256 × 160, FFT).

airways resistance (104% vs. 93%, respectively) and elastance (21% vs. 27%, respectively). The white and red lines in the figure outline the lung contour before and after the Methacholine inhalation (MCh) challenge, respectively. Airway resistance and tissue elastance were measured immediately following each scan. Lung images were then analyzed using local standard deviation (SD) in sliding (9 × 9 pixels^2) ROIs. The ventilation heterogeneity index (*VHI*) was given by:

$$VHI\ (\%) = \frac{SD_{post-MCh} - SD_{pre-MCh}}{SD_{pre-MCh}} x100\% \tag{15}$$

The post-MCh lung function data were normalized by the pre-MCh values to give the percent change. The sham mouse and an OVA mouse data are shown only as an example of the potential X-Centric pre-clinical application. However, data suggested that ventilation heterogeneity following MCh challenge may be commensurate with traditional lung function testing to access the airway hyperresponsiveness in the OVA mouse model. The observed heterogeneity in ventilation distribution could potentially provide a novel endpoint to study disease modification in asthma, as well as for better diagnosis and classification of asthma in the clinic.

The X-Centric method described here should also be beneficial for clinical hyperpolarized lung MRI and other applications where short-TE techniques are

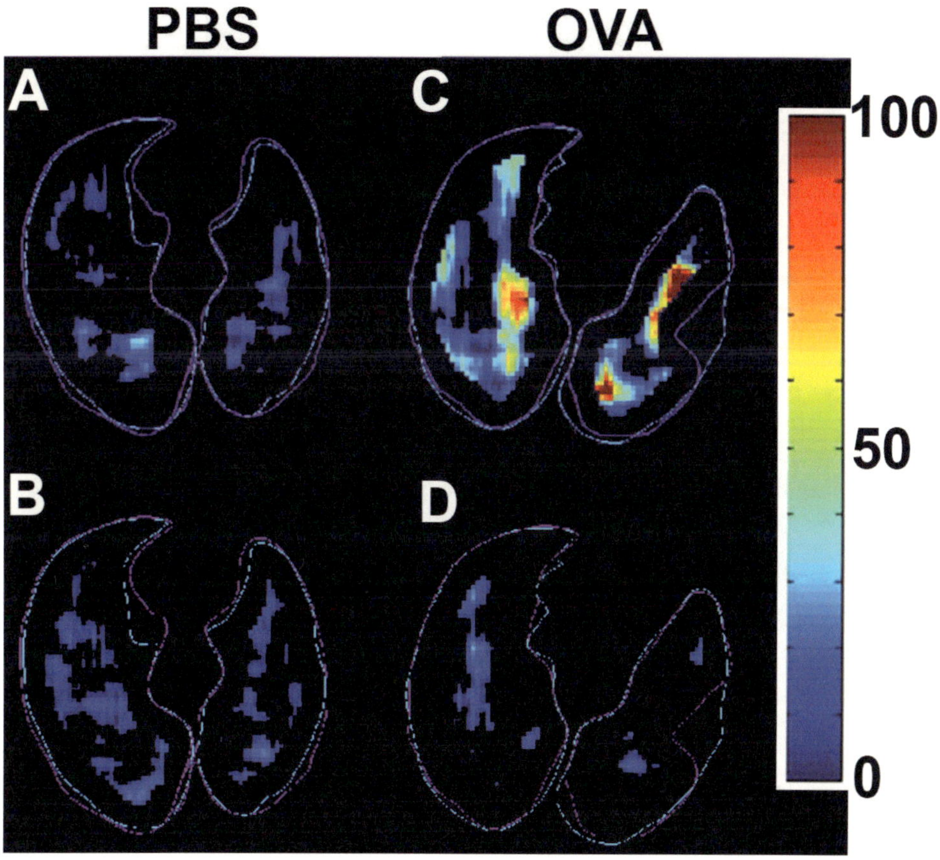

Figure 13.
The VHI maps from a sham mouse (left column) and an OVA treated mouse (right column). The white and red lines in the figure outline the lung contour before and after the Methacholine inhalation challenge, respectively. We applied partial-echo FGRE to acquire a 96 × 48 matrix and zero-filled in phase-encoding direction to get a 96 × 96 matrix using FOV = 2 × 2 cm^2, BW_{read} = 83.3 kHz, TE = 0.42 ms and TR = 1.3 ms. the scan time for each image was ~ 100 ms and the calculated b-value was ~0.7 s/cm^2. The mouse was ventilated at 100 breaths/min and 8.5 ml/kg tidal volume using a ventilation pattern consisting of 160 ms of inhalation, 120 ms of breath-hold (for image acquisition) and 320 ms of exhalation. A series of ^{3}He MR lung images (every 15 s) were acquired before and after methacholine inhalation challenge (160 µg/kg, IV).

needed. **Table 2** helps to estimate the acquisition time for BW_{read} = 62.5 kHz and FOV = 200 × 200 mm^2 (pediatric study [63]) for two matrix sizes frequently used in human studies [6]: 128 × 128 × 14 slices and 256 × 256 × 14 slices (3D case) yielding resolutions of 3.1 × 3.1 × 15 mm^3 and 1.6 × 1.6 × 15 mm^3 at FOV = 400 × 400 × 15mm^3. With the assumption of partial sampling in the phase-encoding direction and taking into account that the maximum strength of the clinical gradient system is typically 4–5 G/cm with a maximum slew rate of 200 T/m/s [6], one can calculate the acquisition to be around 5 s for a 128 × 128 matrix and 16.7 s for a 256 × 256 matrix. As the 256 × 256 matrix at a FOV of 20 × 20 cm^2 corresponds to 781 µm nominal resolution, this should lead to 70% signal decay in airways due to diffusion-weighting according to [22] for the case of full-echo FGRE. The X-Centric approach could eliminate 90% of the signal loss due to incidental diffusion-weighting in the major airways. Parallel imaging approaches [64] or compressed sensing approaches [65, 66] can also speed up data acquisition even more and are a straight-forward extension of the X-Centric approach described here.

Until now, X-Centric has not been used in any pediatric studies; nevertheless, hyperpolarized gas MRI is gradually becoming an important research tool, allowing

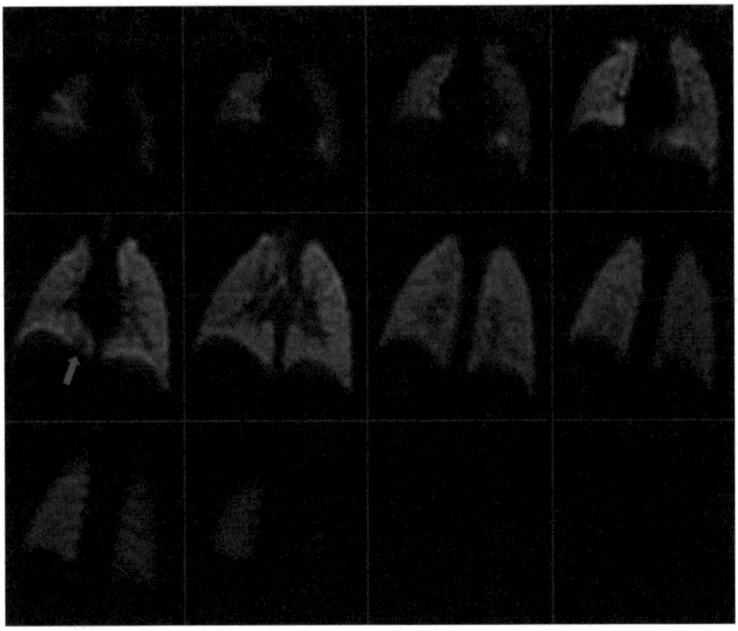

Figure 14.
^{3}He coronal MR images of a 17-month-old non-sedated, unrestrained infant with Cystic Fibrosis. Homogeneous ventilation is seen throughout the lungs. A possible tiny ventilation defect is seen at the right base (arrow). No noticeable motion artifacts are noticeable. 15 spiral interleaved acquisitions (TE = 0.9 ms, TR = 8.1 ms, pixel size = 3 × 3, number of slices = 18; slice thickness = 10 mm, and FOV = 40 × 40 cm^2). Adapted from Altes et al. [28].

for longitudinal observation of lung diseases in children such as Cystic Fibrosis (CF). **Figure 14** shows ^{3}He MRI lung images obtained from a 17-month old patient with CF. Note, the regions of hypo-intensity are difficult to see at this resolution, but using X-Centric, one should be able to gain diagnostic value and better enhance the contrast in these regions. We believe that X-Centric can be very useful for not just CF but the longitudinal observation of other lung diseases like Bronchopulmonary Dysplasia (BPD). Abnormal prematurity at birth (<28 weeks gestation) frequently requires neonatal intensive care and mechanical ventilation due to respiratory distress syndrome due to limited or lack of lung surfactant and incomplete lung development. Ventilator-associated lung injury, along with the extreme prematurity of the lungs themselves, causes abnormal and irregular lung growth (BPD) [67]. The relatively short signal life-time caused by the need to scan newborns inside their neonatal incubators (causing B_0 field distortions, especially at high field) and also the need for smaller FOV make the X-Centric approach ideally suitable for high-resolution neonatal lung MRI.

4. Use of X-centric with other MR-visible nuclei

4.1 Gas phase ^{129}Xe MRI

^{3}He is a rare and expensive isotope (**Table 1**), so a worldwide clinical translation of the ^{3}He MRI method is quite questionable, especially when there is a relatively inexpensive alternative—^{129}Xe MRI. In contrast to the ^{3}He isotope, the ^{129}Xe isotope is much more abundant (~26% natural abundance) and cost efficient (**Table 1**). In addition, recent improvements in the xenon polarization process have enabled sufficient increase in the level of ^{129}Xe polarization (>30%) and production volume of the polarized gas (~2 L per hour) [68, 69]. Presently, ^{129}Xe lung MRI is translating towards a clinical tool, and it has recently been used as a clinical tool (along with ^{3}He MRI) in the United Kingdom [70]. The North-American xenon consortium [71] expects ^{129}Xe MRI to be the Food and Drug Administration approved in the first quarter of 2020.

Presently, the main directions of ^{3}He MRI are pediatric and neonatal studies (using relatively small doses of ^{3}He) mainly due to the cost of the ^{3}He isotope and the high quality of the ^{3}He lung images. In turn, ^{129}Xe MRI is much more suited for adult lung imaging; however, the low SNR of ^{129}Xe images (compared to ^{3}He) impede the development of many novel acquisition schemes that are highly sensitive to SNR [72], such as isotropic voxel static-ventilation imaging and accelerated multiple *b*-value diffusion-weighting MRI [73]. Mentioned above, recent improvement in xenon polarization [68, 69] provides a way to develop advanced imaging methods previously not possible. This is especially critical for investigations in patients with asthma and COPD. Here we report the isotropic-voxel, high-resolution 3D ^{129}Xe static-ventilation image acquired in a single 16 s breath-hold, with the necessary and sufficient SNR to quantify ventilation defect percent [74] estimates (an efficient asthma and COPD biomarker). To the best of our knowledge, a voxel size of 3 × 3 × 3 mm^3 is the highest currently achieved resolution for ^{129}Xe human lung images. **Figures 15** and **16** show the axial and coronal lung images obtained for a healthy volunteer using an isotropic voxel 3D FGRE pulse sequence. The central slice SNR was around 30 for both axial and coronal view images. The gas phase of ^{129}Xe has a relatively low free diffusion coefficient (0.14 cm^2/s in air,

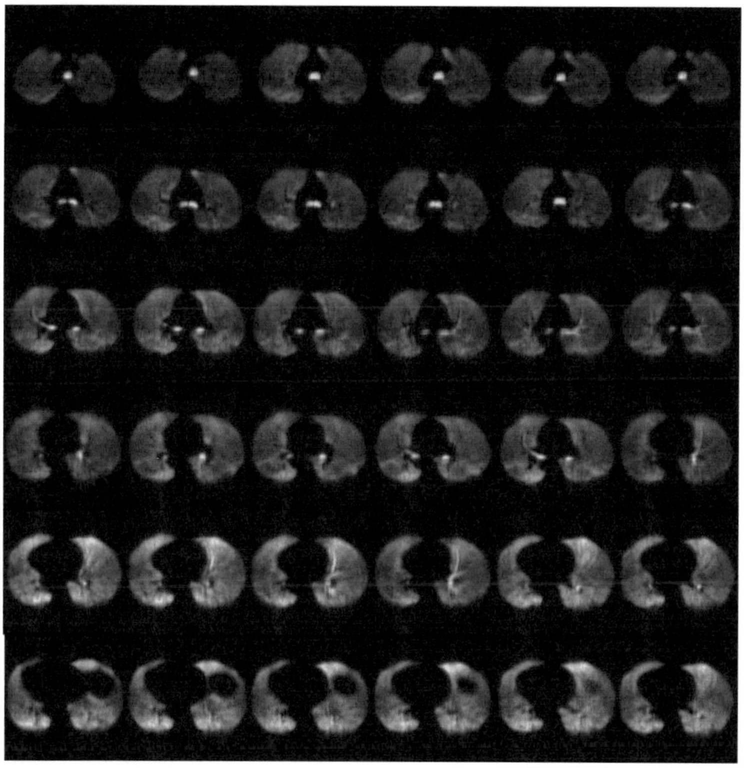

Figure 15.
Axial view isotropic ^{129}Xe MRI static-ventilation slices from superior to inferior for a healthy volunteer. Isotropic-voxel ^{129}Xe static-ventilation images were acquired using an axial plane 3D fast gradient-recalled Echo sequence (TE/TR/initial-flip-angle = 1.3 ms/4.0 ms/0.9°, variable-flip-angle, reconstructed matrix size = 128 × 128 × 104 [axial view], pixel bandwidth = 217 Hz, and FOV = 40 × 40 × 32 cm^3, voxel size = 3 × 3 × 3 mm^3). ^{129}Xe lung images by and courtesy of G. Parraga.

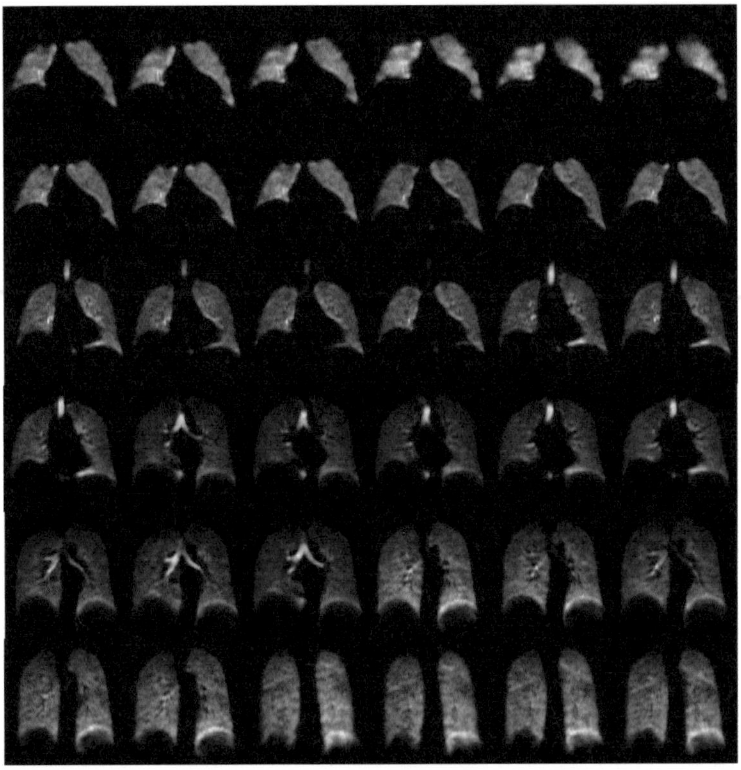

Figure 16.
Coronal view isotropic ^{129}Xe MRI static-ventilation slices from anterior to posterior for a healthy volunteer. Isotropic-voxel ^{129}Xe static-ventilation images were acquired using an axial plane 3D fast gradient-recalled Echo sequence (TE/TR/initial-flip-angle = 1.3 ms/4.0 ms/0.9°, variable-flip-angle, reconstructed matrix size = 128 × 128 × 104 [axial view], pixel bandwidth = 217 Hz, and FOV = 40 × 40 × 32 cm^3, voxel size = 3 × 3 × 3 mm^3). ^{129}Xe lung images by and courtesy of G. Parraga.

Table 1) and relatively long signal life-time (10–30 ms depends on the field strength [75]), so the benefits of the X-Centric approach (overcoming a high diffusivity and short T_2*), may not be very obvious for the case of healthy subjects compared to the traditional FGRE sequence. However, lungs of patients with severe emphysema, COPD (smokers or ex-smokers), BPD and Alpha-1 Antitrypsin Deficiency may show regions with significant terminal airways destruction, changing the diffusion regime to nearly-free diffusion (xenon $D \approx 0.22$ cm^2/s when mixed 50/50 with helium-4 [6]) in such regions, naturally leading to substantial local reduction of T_2* (up to 50% reduction due to the fast motion through the local B_o inhomogeneities within the lung airspaces) [73] especially at high field. X-Centric, is a short-TE method that should be able to better visualize lung regions with short T_2*; and therefore, a better tool for helping to make clinical decisions and for therapy planning.

4.2 Dissolved phase ^{129}Xe MRI

Unlike its counterpart ^{3}He, ^{129}Xe is highly soluble in a variety of solvents and biological materials, and exhibits a large range of chemical shifts within these distinct chemical environments (Ostwald solubility coefficients of 0.17 [40]). Of particular interest is dissolved phase ^{129}Xe residing in and exchanging with lung tissue (tissue barrier) and red blood cells (RBC) [76–78]. The exchange can be measured using MRI and it is also possible distinctly resolve and quantify ^{129}Xe within the tissue barrier and RBC. Exploiting these signals for diagnostic imaging purposes can be difficult since for example, only about 2% of inhaled xenon dissolves into the tissue barrier and RBC [76, 79], and the corresponding T_2^* values are often short (~2 ms) [80]. There is an urgent need for efficient short-TE methods to acquire these short T_2^* signals and enable deeper study of a number of lung abnormalities such as ventilation/perfusion mismatch [81, 82] and of other organs including xenon brain perfusion imaging [72, 83] and imaging of the xenon-encapsulated Cryptophane-A functionalized with anti-cancer drugs [84].

The feasibility of the X-centric method was initially demonstrated using ^{3}He for high-resolution rat lung imaging [39] indicating its ability to overcome diffusion induced signal attenuation within the trachea and substantially reducing TE and t_d as well as the magnitude of the imaging gradient [27]. The low diffusivity and low gyromagnetic ratio of ^{129}Xe (**Table 1**) suggest that diffusion decay due to the imaging gradients would not be an obstacle for high-resolution ^{129}Xe gas MRI; however, the relatively short T_2^* of the dissolved xenon remains a problem, as it leads to signal decay and contributes to image blurring simultaneously. Clearly, short-TE pulse sequences such as spiral [85, 86] or X-Centric [17, 27] are absolutely necessary to acquire images of xenon dissolved in lung tissue and blood.

Figure 17b shows dissolved phase hyperpolarized xenon obtained from within a water-filled resolution phantom (**Figure 17a**) on a clinical 3 T MRI scanner (maximum gradient strength was 5 G/cm, sequence parameters are shown in **Table 2**). The ^{129}Xe image shows that X-Centric can be used to image dissolved phase xenon efficiently (within a breath-hold) and with reasonable signal-to-noise ratio (SNR = 12). After reconstruction, the smallest geometric features of the resolution phantom in the X-Centric image are discernable (yellow arrows). It should be noted, that the available SNR achievable when imaging dissolved phase ^{129}Xe principally depends on concentration, polarization and relaxation times and even physiological parameters such as blood flow and blood oxygenation. The quality of the polarizer, solubility of the solvents used and chemical environments all play a role. Nevertheless, techniques employing significant reductions in echo-times can deliver higher SNR than is typically achievable for spins within environments where their transverse relaxation times are significantly shortened. Though, the phantom dissolved-phase spins had estimated T_2^*-values of roughly 20 ms, the potential for using X-Centric for imaging xenon within the tissue barrier, RBC and

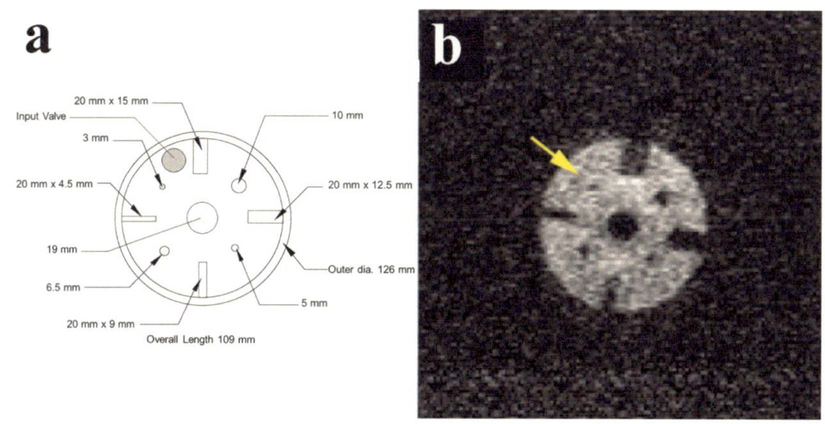

Figure 17.
*Resolution phantom (a) and (b) ^{129}Xe X-centric image obtained in a clinical 3 T MRI scanner. Signal-to-noise ratio value was 12.5. The yellow arrow indicates the 3 mm diameter feature of the resolution phantom demonstrating resolution of the smallest feature of the phantom. The X-centric sequence parameters are shown in **Table** 2. Adapted from Ouriadov et al. [17].*

brain ($T_2^* < 2$ ms) is high and the prospects for high-resolution dissolved phase imaging (currently not available) are demonstrated.

4.3 Static-ventilation ^{19}F MRI

The limited use of the hyperpolarized $^{3}He/^{129}Xe$ MRI imaging modality can be partially explained by its need for utilizing expensive isotopes and polarizers, the latter requiring specially-trained personnel. Inert inhaled fluorinated gas MRI can be a promising and less expensive (**Table 1**) alternative to hyperpolarized $^{3}He/^{129}Xe$ MRI. ^{19}F MRI does not require the use of rare isotopes (100% naturally abundant, **Table 1**) or expensive polarizers. ^{19}F gases (such as perfluoropropane (C_3F_8) and sulfur hexafluoride (SF_6) [17, 18]) can be imaged using high field (≥1.5 T) clinical MRI scanners; however, a multi-nuclear amplifier and receiver along with RF coils tuned to the ^{19}F frequency are still required [18, 19]. Fluorine-19 has a large gyromagnetic ratio (~95% of ^{1}H, **Table 1**), both SF_6 and C_3F_8 have several ^{19}F atoms per molecule, and have relatively short T_1 values making these highly attractive options for researchers (**Table 1**, [87]). Short T_1 translates to overcoming their low thermal polarization [17, 88] values by rapid signal averaging. Additionally, because it is not hyperpolarized, Fluorine-19 gases can be mixed with O_2 without polarization losses, preserving the image quality patient safety simultaneously during a breath-hold scan [89]. Inert fluorinated gases have very short T_2^* values ($T_2^* < 2$ ms [87]), therefore imaging methods with short echo times are preferable. As we demonstrated previously, the X-Centric acquisition can be reliably used for phantom and *in-vivo* measurements using both ^{3}He and ^{129}Xe gases. Similar to the dissolved ^{129}Xe case, a short apparent transverse relaxation time specific to the fluorinated gas can potentially lead to fast signal attenuation and image blurring. As X-Centric is a short-TE sequence it should be able to ensure sufficient SNR of the fluorinated gas images, and also minimal image blurring. **Figure 18a** and **b** show an SF_6 high-resolution phantom (**Figure 14a**) and rat lung images obtained using X-Centric on a clinical 3 T MRI scanner (maximum gradient strength was 5 G/cm, *in-vivo* image sequence parameters are shown in **Table 2**). *In-vivo* data acquisition was synchronized to breath-hold durations using the ventilator [17]. Rat lungs were saturated with an SF_6/O_2 80/20 gas mixture during 3 min of normal free breathing at a breathing rate of 60 breaths/min. After 3 min, the fluorinated gas/O_2 mixture was suspended followed by a 10 sec breath-hold to obtain *in-vivo* rat lung image (**Figure 18b**) [17]. Inert fluorinated gas images confirm that X-Centric ensures

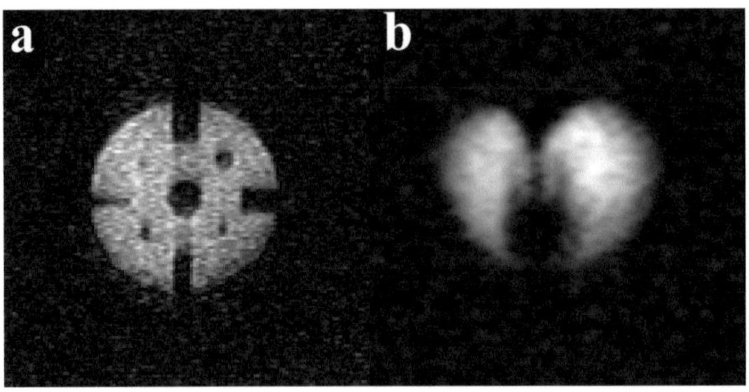

Figure 18.
*(a) An SF_6-filled resolution phantom image (FOV = 20 × 20 cm^2, BW_{read} = 200 Hz/pixel) obtained using X-centric (TE = 0.5 ms, SNR = 14) and (b) in-vivo ^{19}F X-centric rat lung image obtained in a clinical 3 T MRI scanner. SNR values were 14 and 40 respectively. ^{19}F X-centric sequence parameters are shown in **Table 2**. Figure adapted from Ouriadov et al. [17].*

sufficient SNR (14 and 40 for the phantom and *in-vivo* images respectively) and resolution (phantom images shows all details) of fluorinated gas images, when apparent transverse relaxation time is less than 2 ms. These results suggest the possibility for translating these techniques directly to human use because they are demonstrated using a clinical scanner using clinical gradient coils.

4.4 Dynamic ${}^{19}F$ MRI

${}^{19}F$ gas MRI also has a high potential for successful dynamic lung imaging [88, 90] due to the fact that fluorinated gases can be mixed with O_2 which helps to restore the initial magnetization faster (decreasing T_1), in contrast to the hyperpolarized gases. Furthermore, imaging times are shortened and breath-holds are more easily tolerated by the patients [89]. A technique like this permits the acquisition of regional fractional-ventilation [23, 48, 91] which can be very useful as a radiation free alternative to CT for detecting gas trapping in lung diseases such as lung fibrosis and COPD [88]. Recently, free-breathing ${}^{19}F$ (C_3F_8) dynamic lung imaging has been demonstrated in human lungs [89]. **Figure 19** (top panel) shows the gradual wash-out ${}^{19}F$ gas within the ${}^{19}F$ MRI lung images obtained from a COPD patient for eight wash-out breaths [89]. As expected, each new wash-out breath of air replaced some volume of the fluorinated gas in lung, so the signal intensity of the resulting images was gradually attenuated. The following equation can be fitted to this wash-out data [48]:

$$S(n) = S_0 \cdot (1 - r)^n \tag{16}$$

where S_0 is the initial signal, n is the breath number, $S(n)$ is the signal intensity after a certain number of wash-out breaths and r is the fractional-ventilation parameter [17, 48]. In turn, r can be expressed as the fraction between new ${}^{19}F$ incoming to lung, and the total volume of ${}^{19}F$ (V_{total}) [17, 48]:

$$r = \frac{V_{new}}{V_{total}} = \frac{V_{new}}{V_{old} + V_{new}} \tag{17}$$

where V_{new} and V_{old} are the "new" and "old" gas volumes in each voxel at each breath. In general, Eq. (16) can be approximated with the stretched exponential (or Kohlrausch) function [92]:

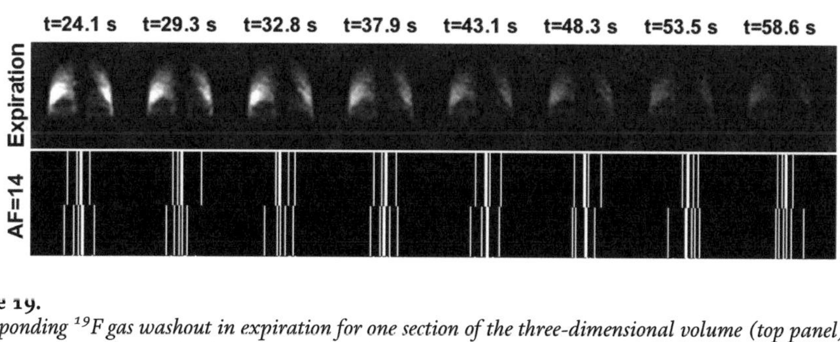

Figure 19.
Corresponding ${}^{19}F$ gas washout in expiration for one section of the three-dimensional volume (top panel). ${}^{19}F$ washout was started at 24.6 s. Images were acquired using a coronal plane 3D spoiled gradient-Echo sequence (TE/TR/flip-angle = 1 ms/3 ms/5°, matrix size = 192 × 130 × 88, pixel bandwidth = 550 Hz, and FOV = 50 × 37.5 × 35.2 cm³, voxel size = 2.6 × 2.9 × 4 mm³) with a generalized auto-calibrating partially parallel acquisition with a reduction factor of 2 in a single breath-hold. Figure adapted from Gutberlet et al. [89]. Sparsity pattern for AF = 14 (bottom panel) depicting the k-space under-sampling scheme, ensuring a variety of sparsity patterns for each time point or wash-out breath. AF = accelaration factor.

$$S(n) = \exp\left[(-nr)^{\beta}\right] \tag{18}$$

where $0 < \beta \leq 1$, and r is the fractional-ventilation. This simple function has been recently used to combine the CS method with under-sampling in the parametric direction [93], which permitted an acceleration factor (AF) of 7 in multi b-value diffusion-weighted ^{3}He MRI measurements [73]. Generally, a reasonable choice of the AF value depends on a number of the images in parametric direction. The main idea behind this relationship is to keep the reconstruction errors low [93]. As we stated above in this chapter, X-Centric is Cartesian pulse sequence, which can be naturally used for under-sampling in imaging (phase-encoding) and parametric (time) directions following CS with the stretched exponential method [93]. To our knowledge this is first record of the possibility of using CS combined with the stretched exponential method for dynamic lung imaging studies. **Figure 19** (bottom panel) shows an under-sampled X-Centric k-space pattern ensuring AF = 14. Remarkably, this means that only 8% of k-space, or five k-space lines (out of 64) are sampled to achieve a "full dataset" and each image in time can be acquired 13 times faster, which obviously helps to avoid the motion artifacts common to free-breathing data acquisition. Additionally, X-Centric can potentially ensure a much shorter TE compared to the spoiled gradient-echo sequence (TE = 1 ms) used to obtained ^{19}F human lung images [89]. Retrospective X-Centric-like under-sampling of the ^{19}F dynamic rat lung *in-vivo* data (64×64 matrix size, nine wash-out images [17]) available to us has confirmed that AF = 14 led to less than a 12% reconstruction difference (pixel-by-pixel comparison between the fully-sampled image and one reconstructed from the retrospectively under-sampled k-space). Therefore, the choice of X-Centric for dynamic ^{19}F gas MRI lung imaging will speed up imaging time and improve image quality making it an optimal choice for this kind of imaging.

The remaining obstacle preventing wide-spread high-resolution ^{19}F MRI with or without X-Centric is the generally low SNR of ^{19}F lung images. In this particular case, the further improvement of the image quality strongly depends on a hardware component, specifically from RF coil systems. It has been recently demonstrated that the use of a multi-channel phased-receive array can significantly improve the image quality of the ^{19}F MRI lung images [94]. This is a very promising result suggesting that the combination of the X-Centric method with advanced array-type RF coil system will permit future high-resolution ^{19}F MRI human lung imaging in both static-ventilation and dynamic studies.

5. Conclusion

In summary, hyperpolarized ^{3}He X-Centric MR imaging with high spatial resolution was proven to be a robust technique in phantom and mouse lung measurements yielding a nominal resolution of 39 μm and 78 μm respectively. In particular, mouse major airways with less restricted diffusion of ^{3}He ($D \sim 0.9$ cm^2/s) could only be visualized with the X-Centric method. Note, that the high nominal resolution (78 μm) in *in-vivo* scans was achieved within 1 s breath-hold. These results suggest that the X-Centric method can potentially fill a gap and need for high spatial and temporal resolution imaging method for the small model of asthma studies.

Another beneficial feature of the X-Centric sequence is the significantly reduced echo-time, so the method can be used for imaging of nuclei with short signal life-times such as hyperpolarized ^{129}Xe dissolved within the lung tissue barrier and/or

Red Blood Cells, and inert fluorinated gas (SF_6) inside the lungs. In both cases the T_2* value is less than 2 ms. The feasibility and future potential of short-TE X-Centric-based X-Nuclei measurements were demonstrated using ^{129}Xe dissolved in water as well as SF_6 within rat lungs.

Acknowledgements

The authors would like to thank the following individuals for assistance with MRI experiments and data analysis: Grace E. Parraga, Giles E. Santyr, Mitchell S. Albert, Marcus J. Couch, Tao Li and Iain K. Ball. A special thanks to Ben T. Chen for providing support for the hyperpolarized ^{3}He gas, animals, and ventilator.

Conflict of interest

The authors do not have any conflict of interest.

Notes/thanks/other declarations

We thank Michael Völker for providing the MatLab code (Projection onto Convex Sets (POCS), 2013) for image reconstruction. We thank Abascal et al. for providing the MatLab code (Signal Decay Into the Reconstruction (SIDER), 2017) for image reconstruction.

Nomenclature

AF	acceleration factor
BW_{read}	bandwidth
BALB/c	laboratory-bred strain of the house mouse
BPD	bronchopulmonary dysplasia
C_3F_8	perfluoropropane
CF	cystic fibrosis
CFA	constant flip angle
COPD	chronic obstructive pulmonary disease
D	self-diffusion coefficient
^{19}F	fluorine-19
FFT	fast Fourier transformation
FGRE	fast gradient recalled echo
FOV	field of view
FWHM	full width at half maximum
GE	general electric
^{1}H	hydrogen-1
^{3}He	helium-3
MCh	methacholine inhalation challenge
MRI	magnetic resonance imaging
O_2	oxygen
OVA	ovalbumin-challenged model
PFR	partial Fourier reconstruction
POCS	projection onto convex sets

RBC	red blood cells
ROI	region of interest
RF	radio frequency
SD	standard deviation
$SD_{post\text{-}MCh}$	post-methacholine challenge SD
$SD_{pre\text{-}MCh}$	pre-methacholine challenge SD
SF6	hexafluoride
SNR	signal to noise ratio
SNR_{nor}	normalized signal to noise ratio
SNR_{theor}	theoretical signal to noise ratio
T_1	longitudinal relaxation time
$T_{1,0}$	T_1 expected in the absence of O_2
T_2^*	apparent transverse relaxation time
T_{scan}	total scan (imaging) time
TE	echo time
T/R	transmit and receive
TR	repetition time
VFA	variable flip angle
VHI	ventilation heterogeneity index
^{129}Xe	xenon-129

Author details

Matthew S. Fox[1,2] and Alexei V. Ouriadov[1,2]*

1 Lawson Health Research Institute, London, ON, Canada

2 Department of Physics and Astronomy, Western University, London, ON, Canada

*Address all correspondence to: aouriado@uwo.ca

References

[1] Albert MS, Cates GD, Driehuys B, Happer W, Saam B, Springer CS, et al. Biological magnetic resonance imaging using laser-polarized 129Xe. Nature. 1994;**370**(6486):199-201

[2] Saam BT, Yablonskiy DA, Kodibagkar VD, Leawoods JC, Gierada DS, Cooper JD, et al. MR imaging of diffusion of 3He gas in healthy and diseased lungs. Magnetic Resonance in Medicine. 2000;**44**(2):174-179

[3] Salerno M, de Lange EE, Altes TA, Truwit JD, Brookeman JR, Mugler JP 3rd. Emphysema: Hyperpolarized helium 3 diffusion MR imaging of the lungs compared with spirometric indexes—Initial experience. Radiology. 2002;**222**(1):252-260

[4] Swift AJ, Wild JM, Fichele S, Woodhouse N, Fleming S, Waterhouse J, et al. Emphysematous changes and normal variation in smokers and COPD patients using diffusion 3He MRI. European Journal of Radiology. 2005; **54**(3):352-358. DOI: 10.1016/j.ejrad.2004.08.002

[5] Evans A, McCormack D, Ouriadov A, Etemad-Rezai R, Santyr G, Parraga G. Anatomical distribution of 3He apparent diffusion coefficients in severe chronic obstructive pulmonary disease. Journal of Magnetic Resonance Imaging. 2007; **26**(6):1537-1547. DOI: 10.1002/jmri.21205

[6] Kirby M, Svenningsen S, Owrangi A, Wheatley A, Farag A, Ouriadov A, et al. Hyperpolarized 3He and 129Xe MR imaging in healthy volunteers and patients with chronic obstructive pulmonary disease. Radiology. 2012; **265**(2):600-610

[7] Altes TA, Powers PL, Knight-Scott J, Rakes G, Platts-Mills TA, de Lange EE, et al. Hyperpolarized 3He MR lung ventilation imaging in asthmatics: Preliminary findings. Journal of Magnetic Resonance Imaging. 2001; **13**(3):378-384. DOI: 10.1002/jmri.1054

[8] de Lange EE, Altes TA, Patrie JT, Gaare JD, Knake JJ, Mugler JP 3rd, et al. Evaluation of asthma with hyperpolarized helium-3 MRI: Correlation with clinical severity and spirometry. Chest. 2006;**130**(4). DOI: 1055-62. DOI 10.1378/chest.130.4.1055

[9] Tzeng YS, Lutchen K, Albert M. The difference in ventilation heterogeneity between asthmatic and healthy subjects quantified using hyperpolarized 3He MRI. Journal of Applied Physiology (Bethesda, MD: 1985). 2009;**106**(3): 813-822. DOI: 10.1152/japplphysiol.01133.2007

[10] Fain SB, Gonzalez-Fernandez G, Peterson ET, Evans MD, Sorkness RL, Jarjour NN, et al. Evaluation of structure-function relationships in asthma using multidetector CT and hyperpolarized He-3 MRI. Academic Radiology. 2008;**15**(6):753-762. DOI: 10.1016/j.acra.2007.10.019

[11] Svenningsen S, Eddy RL, Lim HF, Cox PG, Nair P, Parraga G. Sputum eosinophilia and magnetic resonance imaging ventilation heterogeneity in severe asthma. American Journal of Respiratory and Critical Care Medicine. 2018;**197**(7):876-884. DOI: 10.1164/rccm.201709-1948OC

[12] Hoover DA, Capaldi DP, Sheikh K, Palma DA, Rodrigues GB, Dar AR, et al. Functional lung avoidance for individualized radiotherapy (FLAIR): Study protocol for a randomized, double-blind clinical trial. BMC Cancer. 2014;**14**(1):934. DOI: 10.1186/1471-2407-14-934

[13] Ontario Lung Association. Your Lungs, Your Life: Insights and Solutions to Lung Health in Ontario. 2012:1-24

[14] Canadian Cancer Society. Special topic: Pancreatic cancer. Canadian Cancer Statistics 2017. 2017:1-142

[15] Kovtunov KV, Truong ML, Barskiy DA, Koptyug IV, Coffey AM, Waddell KW, et al. Long-lived spin states for low-field hyperpolarized gas MRI. Chemistry. 2014;**20**(45):14629-14632. DOI: 10.1002/chem.201405063

[16] Kovtunov KV, Romanov AS, Salnikov OG, Barskiy DA, Chekmenev EY, Koptyug IV. Gas phase UTE MRI of propane and propene. Tomography. 2016;**2**(1):49-55. DOI: 10.18383/j.tom.2016.00112

[17] Ouriadov AV, Fox MS, Couch MJ, Li T, Ball IK, Albert MS. In vivo regional ventilation mapping using fluorinated gas MRI with an x-centric FGRE method. Magnetic Resonance in Medicine. 2015;**74**(2):550-557. DOI: 10.1002/mrm.25406

[18] Couch MJ, Ball IK, Li T, Fox MS, Littlefield SL, Biman B, et al. Pulmonary ultrashort echo time 19F MR imaging with inhaled fluorinated gas mixtures in healthy volunteers: Feasibility. Radiology. 2013;**269**(3):903-909. DOI: 10.1148/radiol.13130609

[19] Halaweish AF, Moon RE, Foster WM, Soher BJ, McAdams HP, MacFall JR, et al. Perfluoropropane gas as a magnetic resonance lung imaging contrast agent in humans. Chest. 2013; **144**(4):1300-1310. DOI: 10.1378/chest.12-2597

[20] Wang W, Nguyen NM, Yablonskiy DA, Sukstanskii AL, Osmanagic E, Atkinson JJ, et al. Imaging lung microstructure in mice with hyperpolarized 3He diffusion MRI. Magnetic Resonance in Medicine. 2011; **65**(3):620-626. DOI: 10.1002/mrm.22737

[21] Walvick RP, Roche JP, Reno AL, Gounis MJ, Albert MS. Evaluation of oxygen sensitivity of hyperpolarized helium imaging for the detection of pulmonary ischemia. Magnetic Resonance in Medicine. 2016;**75**(5): 2050-2054. DOI: 10.1002/mrm.25714

[22] Driehuys B, Walker J, Pollaro J, Cofer GP, Mistry N, Schwartz D, et al. 3He MRI in mouse models of asthma. Magnetic Resonance in Medicine. 2007; **58**(5):893-900. DOI: 10.1002/mrm.21306

[23] Couch MJ, Ouriadov A, Santyr GE. Regional ventilation mapping of the rat lung using hyperpolarized 129Xe magnetic resonance imaging. Magnetic Resonance in Medicine. 2012;**68**(5): 1623-1631. DOI: 10.1002/mrm.24152

[24] Wild JM, Woodhouse N, Paley MN, Fichele S, Said Z, Kasuboski L, et al. Comparison between 2D and 3D gradient-echo sequences for MRI of human lung ventilation with hyperpolarized 3He. Magnetic Resonance in Medicine. 2004;**52**(3): 673-678. DOI: 10.1002/mrm.20164

[25] Dugas JP, Garbow JR, Kobayashi DK, Conradi MS. Hyperpolarized (3)He MRI of mouse lung. Magnetic Resonance in Medicine. 2004;**52**(6): 1310-1317. DOI: 10.1002/mrm.20300

[26] Mugler JP, Brookeman JR. Method and System for Rapid Magnetic Resonance Imaging of Gases with Reduced Diffusion-Induced Signal Loss. Google Patents; 2006

[27] Ouriadov AV, Santyr GE. High spatial resolution hyperpolarized (3) He MRI of the rodent lung using a single breath X-centric gradient-recalled echo approach. Magnetic Resonance in Medicine. 2017;**78**(6):2334-2341. DOI: 10.1002/mrm.26602

[28] Altes TA, Meyer CH, Mata JF, Froh DK, Paget-Brown A, Gerald Teague W, et al. Hyperpolarized helium-3 magnetic resonance lung imaging of non-sedated

infants and young children: A proof-of-concept study. Clinical Imaging. 2017; **45**:105-110. DOI: 10.1016/j.clinimag.2017.04.004

[29] Bergin CJ, Pauly JM, Macovski A. Lung parenchyma: Projection reconstruction MR imaging. Radiology. 1991;**179**(3):777-781. DOI: 10.1148/radiology.179.3.2027991

[30] Chen BT, Brau AC, Johnson GA. Measurement of regional lung function in rats using hyperpolarized 3helium dynamic MRI. Magnetic Resonance in Medicine. 2003;**49**(1):78-88. DOI: 10.1002/mrm.10336

[31] Viallon M, Berthezene Y, Callot V, Bourgeois M, Humblot H, Briguet A, et al. Dynamic imaging of hyperpolarized3He distribution in rat lungs using interleaved-spiral scans. NMR in Biomedicine. 2000;**13**(4): 207-213. DOI: 10.1002/1099-1492(200006)13:4<207::aid-nbm641>3.0.co;2-g

[32] Salerno M, Altes TA, Brookeman JR, de Lange EE, Mugler JP 3rd. Dynamic spiral MRI of pulmonary gas flow using hyperpolarized (3)He: Preliminary studies in healthy and diseased lungs. Magnetic Resonance in Medicine. 2001; **46**(4):667-677

[33] Gurney PT, Hargreaves BA, Nishimura DG. Design and analysis of a practical 3D cones trajectory. Magnetic Resonance in Medicine. 2006;**55**(3): 575-582. DOI: 10.1002/mrm.20796

[34] Wang JX, Ouriadov A, Stainsby J, Parraga G, Santyr G. 3D hyperpolarized 3He imaging of human lung with isotropic spatial resolution using 3D-cones. In: Proceedings of the 17th Annual Meeting of ISMRM; Stockholm, Sweden. 2009. p. 4601

[35] Zhang Z, Ouriadov AV, Willson C, Balcom BJ. Membrane gas diffusion measurements with MRI. Journal of Magnetic Resonance. 2005;**176**(2): 215-222. DOI: 10.1016/j.jmr.2005.06.009

[36] Shattuck MD, Gewalt SL, Glover GH, Hedlund LW, Johnson GA. MR microimaging of the lung using volume projection encoding. Magnetic Resonance in Medicine. 1997;**38**(6): 938-942

[37] Fox MS, Ouriadov A, Santyr GE. Comparison of hyperpolarized 3He and 129Xe MRI for the measurement of absolute ventilated lung volume in rats. Magnetic Resonance in Medicine. 2014; **71**(3):1130-1136. DOI: 10.1002/mrm.24746

[38] Ouriadov AV, Kennan R, Slipetz D, Santyr G, Williams D, Rutt BK, et al. In-vivo hyperpolarized 3He lung imaging in mice using x-centric fGRE sequence and custom-designed flexivent ventilator. In: Proceedings of the 16th Annual Meeting of ISMRM; Toronto, Canada. 2008. p. 3789

[39] Santyr GE, Lam WW, Parra-Robles JM, Taves TM, Ouriadov AV. Hyperpolarized noble gas magnetic resonance imaging of the animal lung: Approaches and applications. Journal of Applied Physics. 2009;**105**(10):102004. DOI: 10.1063/1.3112143

[40] Moller HE, Chen XJ, Saam B, Hagspiel KD, Johnson GA, Altes TA, et al. MRI of the lungs using hyperpolarized noble gases. Magnetic Resonance in Medicine. 2002; **47**(6):1029-1051. DOI: 10.1002/mrm.10173

[41] Mugler JP 3rd, Altes TA. Hyperpolarized 129Xe MRI of the human lung. Journal of Magnetic Resonance Imaging. 2013;**37**(2):313-331. DOI: 10.1002/jmri.23844

[42] Brown RW, Cheng YCN, Haacke EM, Thompson MR, Venkatesan R. Magnetic Resonance Imaging: Physical

Principles and Sequence Design. 2nd ed. Hoboken, New Jersey: Wiley Blackwell; 2014. DOI: 10.1002/978111 8633953

[43] Foster-Gareau P, Heyn C, Alejski A, Rutt BK. Imaging single mammalian cells with a 1.5 T clinical MRI scanner. Magnetic Resonance in Medicine. 2003; **49**(5):968-971. DOI: 10.1002/ mrm.10417

[44] Chen XJ, Möller HE, Chawla MS, Cofer GP, Driehuys B, Hedlund LW, et al. Spatially resolved measurements of hyperpolarized gas properties in the lung in vivo. Part II: T*2. Magnetic Resonance in Medicine. 1999;**42**(4): 729-737. DOI: 10.1002/(SICI)1522-2594 (199910)42:4<729::AID-MRM15>3.0. CO;2-2

[45] Saam B, Happer W, Middleton H. Nuclear relaxation of ^{3}He in the presence of O_2. Physical Review A. 1995; **52**(1):862-865

[46] Deninger AJ, Eberle B, Ebert M, Grossmann T, Heil W, Kauczor HU, et al. Quantification of regional intrapulmonary oxygen partial pressure evolution during apnea by He-3 MRI. Journal of Magnetic Resonance. 1999; **141**(2):207-216. DOI: 10.1006/ jmre.1999.1902

[47] Ouriadov AV, Lam WW, Santyr GE. Rapid 3-D mapping of hyperpolarized 3He spin-lattice relaxation times using variable flip angle gradient echo imaging with application to alveolar oxygen partial pressure measurement in rat lungs. Magma. 2009;**22**(5):309-318. DOI: 10.1007/ s10334-009-0181-3

[48] Santyr GE, Lam WW, Ouriadov A. Rapid and efficient mapping of regional ventilation in the rat lung using hyperpolarized 3He with flip angle variation for offset of RF and relaxation (FAVOR). Magnetic Resonance in Medicine. 2008;**59**(6):1304-1310. DOI: 10.1002/mrm.21582

[49] Nishimura DG. Principles of Magnetic Resonance Imaging. Stanford University; 1996

[50] Chen XJ, Moller HE, Chawla MS, Cofer GP, Driehuys B, Hedlund LW, et al. Spatially resolved measurements of hyperpolarized gas properties in the lung in vivo. Part I: Diffusion coefficient. Magnetic Resonance in Medicine. 1999;**42**(4):721-728. DOI: 10.1002/(SICI)1522-2594(199910)42:4 <721::AID-MRM14>3.0.CO;2-D

[51] Miller G, Altes T, Brookeman J, De Lange E, Mugler Iii J. Hyperpolarized 3He lung ventilation imaging with B 1-inhomogeneity correction in a single breath-hold scan. Magnetic Resonance Materials in Physics, Biology and Medicine. 2004;**16**(5):218-226

[52] Zhao L, Mulkern R, Tseng CH, Williamson D, Patz S, Kraft R, et al. Gradient-echo imaging considerations for hyperpolarized 129Xe MR. Journal of Magnetic Resonance—Series B. 1996; **113**(2):179-183

[53] Stejskal EO, Tanner JE. Spin diffusion measurements: Spin echoes in the presence of a time-dependent field gradient. The Journal of Chemical Physics. 1965;**42**(1):288-292

[54] Danneman PJ, Suckow MA, Brayton C. The Laboratory Mouse. CRC Press; 2012

[55] Chen BT, Yordanov AT, Johnson GA. Ventilation-synchronous magnetic resonance microscopy of pulmonary structure and ventilation in mice. Magnetic Resonance in Medicine. 2005;**53**(1):69-75. DOI: 10.1002/ mrm.20307

[56] Lundblad L, Thompson-Figueroa J, Leclair T, G Irvin C, Bates J. Thoracic gas volume measurements in paralyzed mice. Annals of Biomedical Engineering. 2004;**32**(10):1420-1427. DOI: 10.1114/B: ABME.0000042229.41098.6a

[57] Han H, MacGregor RP, Balcom BJ. Pure phase encode magnetic field gradient monitor. Journal of Magnetic Resonance. 2009;**201**(2):212-217. DOI: 10.1016/j.jmr.2009.09.011

[58] Dominguez-Viqueira W, Ouriadov A, O'Halloran R, Fain SB, Santyr GE. Signal-to-noise ratio for hyperpolarized (3)He MR imaging of human lungs: A 1.5 T and 3 T comparison. Magnetic Resonance in Medicine. 2011;**66**(5): 1400-1404. DOI: 10.1002/mrm.22920

[59] Rose A. The sensitivity performance of the human eye on an absolute scale. Journal of the Optical Society of America. 1948;**38**(2):196-208

[60] Haacke EM, Brown RW, Thompson MR, Venkatesan R. Magnetic Resonance Imaging: Physical Principles and Sequence Design. Magnetic Resonance Imaging: Physical Principles and Sequence Design. New York: NY John Wiley & Sons Ltd; 1999. DOI: 10.1002/ 9781118633953.ch1

[61] Stenger VA, Noll DC, Boada FE. Partial Fourier reconstruction for three-dimensional gradient echo functional MRI: Comparison of phase correction methods. Magnetic Resonance in Medicine. 1998;**40**(3):481-490

[62] Haacke EM, Lindskogj ED, Lin W. A fast, iterative, partial-fourier technique capable of local phase recovery. Journal of Magnetic Resonance (1969). 1991; **92**(1):126-145. DOI: 10.1016/0022-2364 (91)90253-p

[63] Altes TA, Meyer CH, Mata JH, Froh D, Paget-Brown A, Fain S, et al. Hyperpolarized Helium-3 MR imaging of a non-sedated infant: A proof-of-concept study: Preliminary experience. In: Proceedings of the 20th Annual Meeting of ISMRM. Melbourne, Australia; 2012. p. P1355

[64] Chang YV, Quirk JD, Yablonskiy DA. In vivo lung morphometry with accelerated hyperpolarized (3) He diffusion MRI: A preliminary study. Magnetic Resonance in Medicine. 2015; **73**(4):1609-1614. DOI: 10.1002/ mrm.25284

[65] Chan HF, Stewart NJ, Parra-Robles J, Collier GJ, Wild JM. Whole lung morphometry with 3D multiple b-value hyperpolarized gas MRI and compressed sensing. Magnetic Resonance in Medicine. 2017;**77**(5):1916-1925. DOI: 10.1002/mrm.26279

[66] Zhang H, Xie J, Xiao S, Zhao X, Zhang M, Shi L, et al. Lung morphometry using hyperpolarized (129) Xe multi-b diffusion MRI with compressed sensing in healthy subjects and patients with COPD. Medical Physics. 2018;**45**(7):3097-3108. DOI: 10.1002/mp.12944

[67] Westcott A, McCormack DG, Parraga G, Ouriadov A. Advanced pulmonary MRI to quantify alveolar and acinar duct abnormalities: Current status and future clinical applications. Journal of Magnetic Resonance Imaging. 2019;(0):0. DOI: 10.1002/nbm.3165

[68] Norquay G, Collier GJ, Rao M, Stewart NJ, Wild JM. 129Xe-Rb spin-exchange optical pumping with high photon efficiency. Physical Review Letters. 2018;**121**(15): 153201. DOI: 10.1103/ PhysRevLett.121.153201

[69] Goodson BM, Ranta K, Skinner JG, Coffey AM, Nikolaou P, Gemeinhardt M, et al. Chapter 2—The physics of hyperpolarized gas MRI A2. In: Albert MS, Hane FT, editors. Hyperpolarized and Inert Gas MRI. Boston: Academic Press; 2017. pp. 23-46. DOI: 10.1016/ B978-0-12-803675-4.00002-6

[70] Wild JM, Collier G, Marshall H, Smith L, Norquay G, Swift AJ, et al. P283 hyperpolarised gas MRI—A pathway to Clinical diagnostic imaging. Thorax. 2015;**70**(Supp. 3):

A220.3-A220A1. DOI: 10.1136/thoraxjnl-2015-207770.419

[71] 129Xe MRI Clinical Trials Consortium. [Internet]. 2018. https://cpircchmcorg/XeMRICTC.

[72] Rao MR, Stewart NJ, Griffiths PD, Norquay G, Wild JM. Imaging human brain perfusion with inhaled hyperpolarized 129Xe MR imaging. Radiology. 2018;**286**(2):659-665. DOI: 10.1148/radiol.2017162881

[73] Westcott A, Guo F, Parraga G, Ouriadov A. Rapid single-breath hyperpolarized Noble gas MRI based biomarkers of airspace enlargement. Journal of Magnetic Resonance Imaging. 2018;**2018**. DOI: 10.1002/jmri.26574

[74] Svenningsen S, Kirby M, Starr D, Leary D, Wheatley A, Maksym GN, et al. Hyperpolarized (3) He and (129) Xe MRI: Differences in asthma before bronchodilation. Journal of Magnetic Resonance Imaging. 2013; **38**(6):1521-1530. DOI: 10.1002/jmri.24111

[75] Xu X, Norquay G, Parnell SR, Deppe MH, Ajraoui S, Hashoian R, et al. Hyperpolarized 129Xe gas lung MRI-SNR and T2* comparisons at 1.5 T and 3 T. Magnetic Resonance in Medicine. 2012;**68**(6):1900-1904. DOI: 10.1002/mrm.24190

[76] Mugler JP, Driehuys B, Brookeman JR, Cates GD, Berr SS, Bryant RG, et al. MR imaging and spectroscopy using hyperpolarized 129Xe gas: Preliminary human results. Magnetic Resonance in Medicine. 1997;**37**(6):809-815. DOI: 10.1002/mrm.1910370602

[77] Sakai K, Bilek AM, Oteiza E, Walsworth RL, Balamore D, Jolesz FA, et al. Temporal dynamics of hyperpolarized 129Xe resonances in living rats. Journal of Magnetic Resonance. Series B. 1996;**111**(3): 300-304

[78] Ruppert K, Brookeman JR, Hagspiel KD, Driehuys B, Mugler JP. NMR of hyperpolarized129Xe in the canine chest: Spectral dynamics during a breath-hold. NMR in Biomedicine. 2000;**13**(4):220-228. DOI: 10.1002/1099-1492(200006)13:4<220::aid-nbm638>3.0.co;2-f

[79] Kaushik SS, Robertson SH, Freeman MS, He M, Kelly KT, Roos JE, et al. Single-breath clinical imaging of hyperpolarized (129)Xe in the airspaces, barrier, and red blood cells using an interleaved 3D radial 1-point Dixon acquisition. Magnetic Resonance in Medicine. 2016;**75**(4):1434-1443. DOI: 10.1002/mrm.25675

[80] Driehuys B, Cofer GP, Pollaro J, Mackel JB, Hedlund LW, Johnson GA. Imaging alveolar–capillary gas transfer using hyperpolarized 129Xe MRI. Proceedings of the National Academy of Sciences. 2006;**103**(48):18278-18283. DOI: 10.1073/pnas.0608458103

[81] Fox MS, Ouriadov A, Thind K, Hegarty E, Wong E, Hope A, et al. Detection of radiation induced lung injury in rats using dynamic hyperpolarized (129)Xe magnetic resonance spectroscopy. Medical Physics. 2014;**41**(7):072302. DOI: 10.1118/1.4881523

[82] Doganay O, Matin T, Chen M, Kim M, McIntyre A, McGowan DR, et al. Time-series hyperpolarized xenon-129 MRI of lobar lung ventilation of COPD in comparison to V/Q-SPECT/CT and CT. European Radiology. 2018. DOI: 10.1007/s00330-018-5888-y

[83] Mazzanti ML, Walvick RP, Zhou X, Sun Y, Shah N, Mansour J, et al. Distribution of hyperpolarized xenon in the brain following sensory stimulation: Preliminary MRI findings. PLoS One. 2011;**6**(7):e21607. DOI: 10.1371/journal.pone.0021607

[84] Zeng Q, Guo Q, Yuan Y, Yang Y, Zhang B, Ren L, et al. Mitochondria

targeted and intracellular biothiol triggered hyperpolarized (129)Xe magnetofluorescent biosensor. Analytical Chemistry. 2017;**89**(4): 2288-2295. DOI: 10.1021/acs. analchem.6b03742

[85] Zanette B, Stirrat E, Jelveh S, Hope A, Santyr G. Physiological gas exchange mapping of hyperpolarized (129) Xe using spiral-IDEAL and MOXE in a model of regional radiation-induced lung injury. Medical Physics. 2018; **45**(2):803-816. DOI: 10.1002/mp.12730

[86] Doganay O, Wade T, Hegarty E, McKenzie C, Schulte RF, Santyr GE. Hyperpolarized (129) Xe imaging of the rat lung using spiral IDEAL. Magnetic Resonance in Medicine. 2016;**76**(2): 566-576. DOI: 10.1002/mrm.25911

[87] Chang YV, Conradi MS. Relaxation and diffusion of perfluorocarbon gas mixtures with oxygen for lung MRI. Journal of Magnetic Resonance. 2006; **181**(2):191-198. DOI: 10.1016/j. jmr.2006.04.003

[88] Couch MJ, Fox MS, Viel C, Gajawada G, Li T, Ouriadov AV, et al. Fractional ventilation mapping using inert fluorinated gas MRI in rat models of inflammation and fibrosis. NMR in Biomedicine. 2016;**29**(5):545-552. DOI: 10.1002/nbm.3493

[89] Gutberlet M, Kaireit TF, Voskrebenzev A, Lasch F, Freise J, Welte T, et al. Free-breathing dynamic (19)F gas MR imaging for mapping of regional lung ventilation in patients with COPD. Radiology. 2018;**286**(3): 1040-1051. DOI: 10.1148/ radiol.2017170591

[90] Couch MJ, Ouriadov AV, Albert MS. Chapter 18—Pulmonary imaging using 19f mri of inert fluorinated gases. In: Hyperpolarized and Inert Gas MRI. Boston: Academic Press; 2017. pp. 279-292. DOI: 10.1016/B978-0-12-803675-4.00018-X

[91] Deninger AJ, Månsson S, Petersson JS, Pettersson G, Magnusson P, Svensson J, et al. Quantitative measurement of regional lung ventilation using 3He MRI. Magnetic Resonance in Medicine. 2002;**48**(2): 223-232. DOI: 10.1002/mrm.10206

[92] Berberan-Santos MN, Bodunov EN, Valeur B. Mathematical functions for the analysis of luminescence decays with underlying distributions 1. Kohlrausch decay function (stretched exponential). Chemical Physics. 2005; **315**(1–2):171-182. DOI: 10.1016/j. chemphys.2005.04.006

[93] Abascal JFPJ, Desco M, Parra-Robles J. Incorporation of Prior Knowledge of the Signal Behavior into the Reconstruction to Accelerate the Acquisition of MR Diffusion Data. ArXiv e-prints [Internet]. 2017; 1702. Available from: http://adsabs.harvard.ed u/abs/2017arXiv170202743A

[94] Charles C, Jones2 RW, Halaweish AF, Ainslie MD. Parallel imaging for short breath hold times in perfluorinated gas imaging of the lung [abstract]. In: Proceedings of the 23rd Annual Meeting of ISMRM; Toronto, Canada. 2015. p. 3984

Section 5

Uses of MRI in Radiotherapy

Chapter 6

4D-MRI in Radiotherapy

Chunhao Wang and Fang-Fang Yin

Abstract

Four-dimensional (4D) imaging provides a useful estimation of tissue motion pattern and range for radiation therapy of moving targets. 4D-CT imaging has been a standard care of practice for stereotactic body radiation therapy of moving targets. Recently, 4D-MRI has become an emerging developmental area in radiotherapy. In comparison with 4D-CT imaging, 4D-MRI provides better spatial rendering of radiotherapy targets in abdominal and pelvis regions with improved visualization of soft tissue motion. Successful implementation of 4D-MRI requires an integration of optimized acquisition protocols, advanced image reconstruction techniques, and sufficient hardware capabilities. The proposed chapter intends to introduce basic theories, current research, development, and applications of 4D-MRI in radiotherapy.

Keywords: 4D-MRI, radiotherapy, image reconstruction, respiratory motion, motion artifacts

1. Introduction

The role of modern radiotherapy in cancer treatment is to irradiate target volumes that contain disease sites while sparing surrounding normal tissue. In classic 3D-based radiotherapy, treatment volumes are typically defined in **Figure 1(a)**. Gross tumor volume (GTV) contains the primary tumor or malignant tissue, and clinical target volume (CTV) contains GTV plus its surrounding tissue that may have subclinical disease that cannot be definitely revealed by medical imaging (though it is uncommon that CTV is identical to GTV in certain definitive radiotherapy). Planning target volume (PTV), which is often defined as treatment volume in a radiotherapy plan, is defined as CTV plus a margin that accounts for possible tissue displacement and patient positioning uncertainty within a treatment course that may last several weeks [1, 2]. This CTV to PTV margin can be called as setup margin. Depending on different treatment sites and disease stage, setup margin ranges from a few millimeters to 1–2 cm. However, in some radiotherapy treatment, the GTV volume is not stable: when treating tumors in lung, esophagus, and abdominal regions (liver, pancreas, etc.), tumors move under the effect of respiratory activity. Such target motion, referred as respiratory motion, has to be accounted in radiotherapy for effective therapeutic outcome. Thus, a large setup margin for PTV was proposed to account for possible respiratory motion. However, such simple solution has two problems: (1) amplitudes of respiratory motion vary among different individuals. Results of 1–2 mm up to 3 cm are commonly observed in clinic. A single large margin may not yield optimal treatment outcome for patients with extended/limited motion amplitudes [3]; and (2) a large setup margin may lead to unnecessary irradiation of normal tissue, which may substantially increase toxicity of radiotherapy. With the

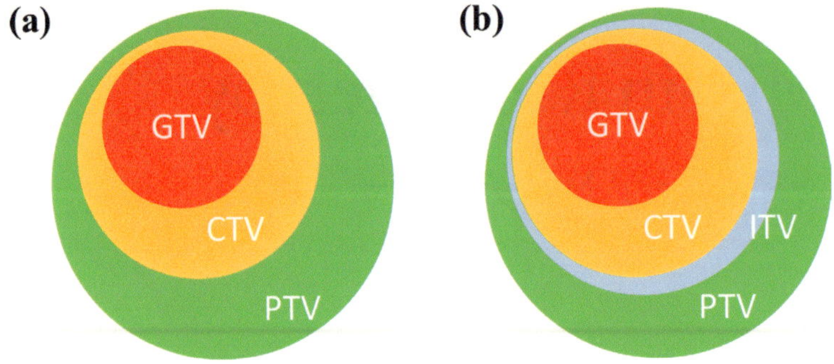

Figure 1.
Diagrams of volume definition in modern radiotherapy. (a) Definitions without consideration of target motion; (b) Definitions with ITV included to account for target motion.

current trend of stereotactic body radiotherapy (SBRT, also referred as stereotactic ablative body radiotherapy SABR) using very high radiation dose to treatment cancer in a few fractions, such big margin with large toxicity becomes unacceptable.

To account for aforementioned issue, dynamic imaging concept was proposed to capture individualized target motion pattern and amplitude. Such information can be used to define an internal target volume (ITV), which adds an internal margin to CTV that accounts for full possible motion range during radiotherapy (**Figure 1(b)**). This internal margin is determined on an individual basis during the initial treatment simulation. Compared to a generous setup margin, the added internal margin can maximize the therapeutic effect while reducing the irradiation to normal tissue [4, 5].

Prior to 4D imaging in radiotherapy, X-ray fluoroscopy imaging using C-arm device was the early effort to determine individualized internal margin [6]. The lack of volumetric information in this approach cannot capture the potential motion pattern heterogeneity. Since CT is the dominant modality for radiotherapy with its irreplaceable tissue electron density information required by radiation dose calculation, proposed in the 2000s, 4D-CT has become the standard imaging technique of treatment moving target [7]. **Figure 2** shows a diagram of 4D-CT. For a simple description, 4D-CT samples projections repetitively at a couch position for at least one respiratory cycle before moving to the next imaging position. With synchronized respiratory cycle information, all projections are retrospectively sorted into

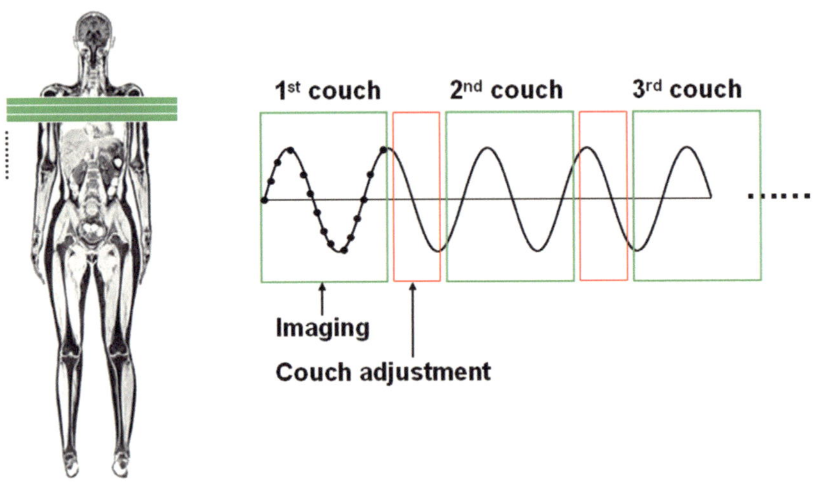

Figure 2.
A simple diagram of 4D-CT implementation.

different phase bins (typically 10) that consists of an averaged respiratory cycle derived from the whole scan period [8]. The respiratory cycle information is usually derived by recording 2D trajectories of external surrogates, such as inferred reflection markers and pneumatic bellows [9, 10]. As a result, multiple 3D CT volumes from different phase volumes are reconstructed. By delineating CTV volumes at each 3D volume, ITV can be generated as a union of CTVs from all phases with a possible small margin for positioning uncertainty.

Despite of its popularity, 4D-CT has a few problems: (1) when patient's breath becomes irregular in terms of amplitude and period length, abrupt changes in projections may lead to motion-induced artifacts in the reconstructed phase volumes. **Figure 3** shows a reconstructed phase volume in 4D-CT. The diaphragm boundary discontinuity with a ghost displacement indicated by red arrow is a typical rendering of motion artifacts in 4D-CT; (2) although trajectories of external surrogates and internal organs are correlated [11], potential hysteresis between the two trajectories may impact overall treatment accuracy [12]; and (3) 4D-CT requires extended scan time and leads to increased imaging radiation dose as a potential patient health risk.

In addition to 4D-CT, ultrasound has been utilized for motion assessment in radiotherapy because of its fast imaging time and relatively simple implementation. Earlier application of ultrasound focused at localizing displaced prostate radiotherapy volume through transrectal imaging [13]. To image respiratory motion, previous work reported its use for upper abdominal radiotherapy. In addition to assess motion at simulation, same imaging strategy can be deployed at each treatment fraction for real-time verification [14, 15]. However, motion assessment using ultrasound sometime can only be achieved by indirect measurement of a nearby landmark instead of target volume [16]. The generally poor visualization capability of ultrasound limits its utilization in the current practice of radiotherapy.

Following the increased utilization of MRI in radiotherapy, 4D-MRI has become a popular area in image-guided radiotherapy (IGRT) after the birth of 4D-CT. Generally, MRI has excellent soft-tissue contrast with zero radiation hazard in comparison to 4D-CT. 4D-MRI is thus highly desirable in the radiotherapy workflow. In the last decade, many works have been done for the development of 4D-MRI. At present, however, there is no fully established 4D-MRI technique by major vendors in radiotherapy clinic. Implementation of 4D-MRI in clinic is still at investigational stage due to excessive technical involvement. Nevertheless, current results of 4D-MRI application showed its promising value in the era of IGRT [17].

In the following section, we will introduce 4D-MRI basic theories and current technologies and discuss emerging topics in 4D-MRI research and development. Radiotherapy application of 4D-MRI will be discussed based on our clinical experience in another section.

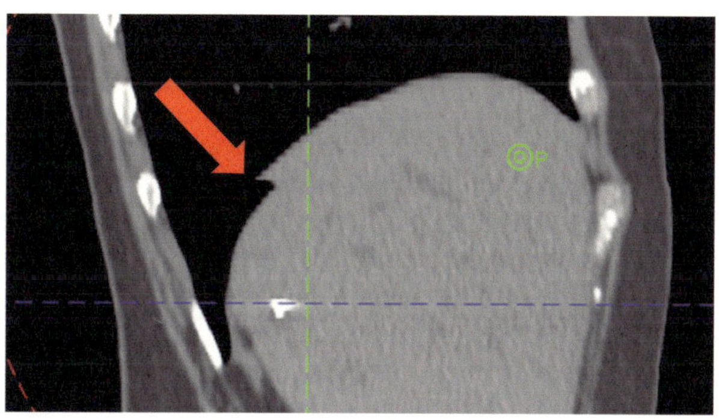

Figure 3.
An example of motion artifacts in 4D-CT.

2. 4D-MRI: basic theories and technologies

In this section, we first describe the brief history of 4D-MRI debut and then discuss basic theories and implementation technologies of current 4D-MRI methods. Frontier research topics in 4D-MRI are introduced in the rear part in this section.

2.1 Fast imaging: early effort

Earliest effort for MRI-based motion quantification focused on 2D-based cine imaging, i.e., continuously acquire images at a fixed 2D coordinate frame. The acquired 2D images could be stacked as a movie that described target motion. This requires fast imaging sequences to achieve high frame rates. Several approaches were employed. Koch et al. first used gradient echo technique in lung motion imaging [18]. Shimizu et al. imaged liver tumor motion with multiple T1-weighted gradient slices [19]. Kirilova et al. used T2-weighted single shot fast spin echo sequence for liver tumor position tracking [20]. A handful of works adopted balanced steady-state free precession (bSSFP) imaging on three orthogonal planes for tumor as well as diaphragm motion tracking [21, 22]. The reported frame rate using bSSFP could be up to 10 frames per second.

The obvious drawback of 2D cine imaging is the deficiency of volumetric motion capture, which is critical when motion pattern is heterogeneous within the imaging region of interest (ROI). Repetitive 3D volume acquisition (i.e., real-time 4D-MRI) was then investigated since it yielded truly real-time volumetric imaging without additional post-processing. This approach is usually accomplished with parallel imaging with a trade of image quality. Blackall et al. used fast file echo with echo planar imaging (FFE-EPI) for real-time 4D-MRI implementation for lung RT planning [23]. In spite of its reported high temporal resolution (up to 330 ms/frame), the acquired image showed considerably less vessel structure details within the lung. Dinkel et al. implemented TREAT sequence, a 3D time-resolved echo shared gradient echo sequence with parallel imaging [24]. This technique achieved a frame rate of 1400 ms/frame covering a large field of view (FOV) (400 × 400 × 300 mm) with a relatively low spatial resolution (voxel size 3.1 × 3.1 × 4 mm). Tryggestad et al. reported their real-time 4D-MRI protocol with frame rate 1000 ms/frame at the cost of lower signal-to-noise ratio (SNR) and intrascan motion [25]. However, these works did not achieve high temporal resolution and acceptable spatial resolution at the same time. Since a typical human's breathing cycle period is about 3–5 seconds, high temporal resolution <500 ms/frame is desired for multiphase reconstruction. In addition, high spatial resolution at the level of 1 mm isotropic voxel size might be necessary for small size SBRT target in lung/liver treatment, which could be 1 cc or less. Currently available MR scanner capabilities limit further improvement of real-time 4D-MRI.

2.2 Retrospective sorting: 2D-based

Retrospective sorting has been the mainstream technique for 4D-MRI reconstruction. Similar to the 4D-CT implementation, retrospective sorting in 4D-MRI records a motion surrogate's trajectory during the scan. Acquisition data are sorted into different bins based on the amplitude/phase information of the surrogate trajectory. To date, retrospective sorting with multislice dynamic 2D acquisition (2D-based sorting) is commonly reported for clinical and preclinical investigations. In short, 2D MRI image slices at interleaved slice locations were sorted accordingly before 3D volume stacking. By theory, this strategy can achieve high spatial resolution while maintaining high in-plane spatial resolution. On the other hand, retrospective sorting requires intensive image post-processing offline with high software demand.

So far, several works of 2D-based sorting techniques have been reported with different motion surrogate selection and image acquisition sequence. von Siebenthal et al. invented a navigator-based sorting method. In this method, navigator slices were acquired at a fixed location, interleaved with slice locations that were sequentially stepped through the imaging volume. 2D images were acquired using 2D bSSFP sequence repetitively for nearly 1 hour. Image sorting was carried based on navigator slice similarity using a cost function that combines directional shifts of image registration [26]. This sophisticated scheme achieve 180 ms/frame temporal resolution and 1.8 × 1.8 mm in-plane resolution, but the navigator acquisition prolonged total scan time and did not guarantee measurement reproducibility.

Remmert et al. investigated the feasibility of using respiratory surrogate. A rapid imaging sequence using 2D fast low-angle shot (FLASH) with generalized auto-calibrating partially parallel acquisition (GRAPPA) was adopted on Cartesian grid. Respiratory surrogate was extracted as the positioning of the piston rod of the imaged dynamic porcine lung phantom [27]. The results demonstrated the feasibility of respiratory surrogate sorting. Hu et al. implemented a respiratory-triggered 4D-MRI reconstruction. The respiratory amplitude was derived from a turbo spin echo sequence, and 2D image acquisition was achieved by T2-weighted EPI [28]. The in vivo demonstration of this technique in healthy volunteers successfully reconstructed four phase volumes.

Other surrogates are also proposed for convenient sorting implementation. Cai et al. proposed a sorting surrogate based on body area (BA), which was defined as the area inside the binary mask of body contour from 2D fast steady-state acquisition (FIESTA). The surrogate trajectory was determined by excluding the low-frequency change of BA as subject anatomic change [29]. Tryggestad et al. integrated signals from Physiologic Monitoring Unit (PMU) by Siemens for retrospective sorting. This PMU signal was derived from a pneumatic device attached to the subject's upper abdomen. Acquired at 50 Hz sampling rate, the PMU signal was synchronized with 2D repetitive acquisition [25].

In spite of its popularity, 2D-based sorting methods suffer from two major problems: (1) large slice thickness (typically 5–10 mm) may not be sufficient to quantify target motion when the target is small, and the reconstructed volume may not look like continuous on slice direction; and (2) the reconstructed images tend to have stitch motion artifacts similar to those in 4D-CT. **Figure 4** shows an example of stitch motion artifacts. This resorting artifact of radiant rays is caused by unpredicted motion change during image acquisition.

2.3 Retrospective sorting: 3D-based

3D-based retrospective sorting has gained its attention with advances of both imaging hardware and software technologies. Similar to 2D-based equivalent, 3D-based retrospective sorting requires motion surrogate recording synchronized with data acquisition. The most distinguished feature of 3D-based sorting is that raw k-space acquisitions, rather than 2D image data in real space, are sorted into different phase volume bins. Image reconstruction in 3D fashion (but could also be done in 2D) has to be performed after retrospective sorting. Image quality can be improved with advanced image reconstruction technique with possible isotropic voxel size. Generally, 3D-based retrospective sorting requires more sophisticated data processing algorithms and more demanding hardware manipulation. Nevertheless, 3D-based retrospective sorting has become the selection by most recent 4D-MRI developments.

In 2008, Tokuda et al. proposed an early trial of 3D-based retrospective sorting. The acquired k-space echo was filled into multiple assigned bins based on

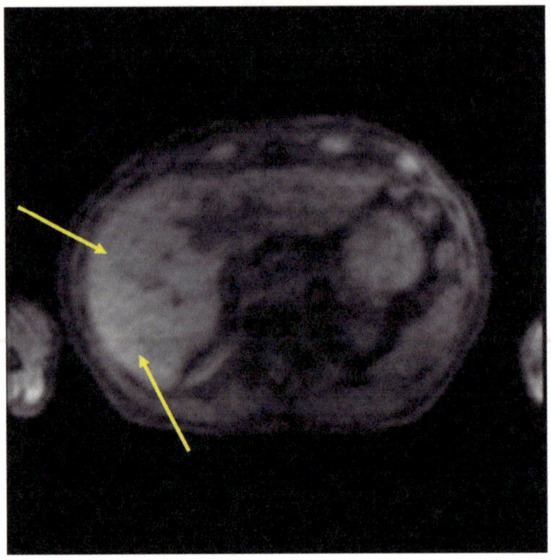

Figure 4.
An example of stitch motion artifacts in reconstructed 4D-MRI. This image was reconstructed from computer simulation instead of human subject imaging.

amplitude ranges of respiratory surrogate, which was implemented by a navigator echo acquired at a configurable sampling rate [30]. In a patient study, 4D volumes were successfully reconstructed using 10.5 min acquisition time with compromised image quality compared with breath-hold (BH) 3D acquisitions.

In the last several years, several representative works with 3D-based sorting have been reported as most recent advances in 4D-MRI. Deng et al. utilized a continuous spoiled gradient echo sequence with 3D radial trajectory for fast volumetric acquisition [31]. Respiratory surrogate was derived as "self-gating" (SG) measurement, which was 1D Fourier transform of SG acquisition lines through the k-space center (k_z direction). Acquisitions were retrospectively sorted into ten phase volumes using phase percentage information on surrogate trajectory, and image reconstruction was carried out with a conjugate-gradient sensitivity encoding (CG-SENSE) with self-sensitivity calibration [32].

Similarly, Feng et al. proposed a 4D-MRI framework XD-GRASP (extra-dimension golden-angle radial sparse parallel) technique, which included 3D radial-based acquisition trajectory and surrogate with SG [33]. Principal component analysis (PCA) could be used on SG surrogate to separate cardiac motion or MR contrast uptake from respiratory motion. Each 3D volume was iteratively reconstructed on radial grid.

Acquisition on Cartesian grid has also been reported. Han et al. invented a rotating 3D Cartesian k-space recording method (ROCK) for 4D-MRI acquisition [34]. This method simulated a quasispiral acquisition trajectory with varying sampling densities on radial direction. Balanced SSFP sequence was chosen for its improved SNR over gradient recalled echo technique, and amplitude-based sorting was based on SG motion surrogate. Wang et al. also implemented a sparse Cartesian-based acquisition trajectory simulating a multi-ray profile regulated by golden-ratio angular increment [35].

2.4 Discussion: technical factors in 4D-MRI

As a summary of current 4D-MRI works (with a focus on 3D-based retrospective sorting approach), we hereby discuss a few key technical factors that one may need to consider for developing a 4D-MRI method:

2.4.1 Acquisition protocol

K-space acquisition can be realized by different techniques since retrospective sorting does not directly depend on data acquisition scheme. Both radial-based and Cartesian-based trajectories are valid for acquisition. Since radial-based trajectories have higher sampling density near k-space center (low-frequency component) in their nature, they might be preferred for fast 3D acquisition. Golden-ratio means or its equivalent technologies are commonly used for 4D-MRI since the azimuthal increments are relatively constant after volume sorting [36–38]. However, radial-based trajectories may lead to severe motion artifacts after retrospective sorting when the subject's motion is irregular [34]. Cartesian-based trajectories could simulate k-space central/peripheral sampling weights in radial-trajectories and might be easier for image reconstruction without data regridding. Nevertheless, both approaches require extensive hardware/software editing that most clinical MR units may not be fully ready for.

To implement SG, low-frequency component in k-space has to be sampled repeatedly during the total acquisition time. As discussed above, SG can be derived as 1D projection on k_z direction through k-space center. SG signal can capture displacement on superior-inferior (SI) direction that is sensitive to respiratory motion [39]. SG can also be derived as phase shift measurement of 0-frequency (DC) point at k-space center [35]. It has to be pointed out that k-space center does not have to be sampled periodically as long as the sampling intervals are known. Since the human breath is mostly modeled as sinusoid waveform, it is more straightforward to sample k-space center at certain rhythms.

2.4.2 Retrospective sorting practice

In retrospective sorting, data binning can use either surrogate's amplitude or phase percentage (temporal location within a breath cycle) information. Both approaches are valid in both 4D-MRI and 4D-CT. However, when the subject's breathing is not regular, potential error could be made in retrospective sorting [40, 41]. In clinical practice, intrascan variation of both breathing amplitude and period is commonly seen. There is no established theory regarding variation theory, but breathing period is subject to more change when the scan time is long for pulmonary function compromised subjects. Drastic change of surrogate amplitude, however, is usually caused by random event such as cough.

To reduce irregularity-induced data divergence, a straightforward way is to employ external motion management devices as in 4D-CT imaging, such as abdominal compression and body vacuum bag. However, such devices can be cumbersome for MR imaging protocols.

During retrospective sorting, one determines certain threshold values and excludes data acquisitions when surrogate trajectory is out of range [29]. In spite of its simplicity, this approach may reduce data utility when the subject's breathing is irregular, which may further lead to undersampling artifacts in the reconstructed images. A soft-gating approach has been reported for amplitude-based on a Gaussian weighting function with its Full width at half maximum (FWHM) determined as a function of surrogate motion range [34]. This approach can improve data utilization with improved SNR in the reconstructed images [42, 43].

Wang et al. designed a spatiotemporal index (STI) as a quadratic sum of amplitude and phase discrepancies in retrospective sorting [35]. Each acquisition can be used for reconstructing multiple phase volumes when discrepancy criteria are met. In combination with the selected acquisition trajectory, such criteria were designed as tight rules near k-space center and loose rules near k-space periphery to further improve data utilization.

2.4.3 Image reconstruction

Image reconstruction has become a focused topic in 4D-MRI because of sparse k-space data after 3D-based retrospective sorting. With the advent of compressed sensing, i.e., extract compressible signal from undersampled data, many iterative MR reconstruction algorithms have been successfully developed [44–46]. In the specific 4D-MRI reconstruction, L1-norm (total variation [47]), L2-norm (total generalized variation, TGV [48]; Tikhonov regularization [49]), and wavelet (Daubechies [50]) regularization algorithms have been utilized. Detailed mathematics of these algorithms go beyond the scope of this discussion.

A unique feature of 4D-MRI reconstruction is the potential implementation of spatiotemporal constrained reconstruction. Because of averaging nature in retrospective sorting, motion continuity is usually guaranteed after reconstructing each phase volume as an independent 3D volume. A possible improvement is view sharing, which enable the use of same data in multiple volumes. Such technique has been widely used in dynamic MRI imaging for pharmacokinetics study [51, 52]. Because of motion sensitivity of low-frequency k-space component, view sharing of high-frequency component in combination with iterative reconstruction is a viable solution [35]. Temporal constraint can also be explicitly written as penalty terms in reconstruction. Total variation representation of finite motion differences has been adopted [33, 34].

2.5 Emerging topics in 4D-MRI research

Trends in 4D-MRI research have been following evolving technologies in radiation oncology. The most relative topic is to use deformable image registration (DIR) to model anatomic motion during respiratory cycles. A detailed description of DIR cannot be included in this section; for a short discussion, DIR tries to wrap one image to another one with much more transform degrees that are different across the ROI instead of 6 rigid transform degrees. A registration is represented by a deformation vector field (DVF) in the same size as the source image, which points each single voxel in source image to its destination in the coordinate system of target image. DIR has been used in radiotherapy for time-series image registration, image outcome for treatment assessment, and dose wrapping for adaptive therapy [53].

In 4D-MRI, the motion-induced anatomic change can be seen as a deformation process. Each phase volume (2D or 3D) is a deformation from a standard reference volume. This reference volume can be a stable phase volume in 4D series (such as end-of-exhalation (EOE) phase) or a breath-hold (BH) volume. Thus, respiratory motion can be described by a series of DVFs derived from DIR. This enables the motion information transfer to recreate respiratory motion derived from one MR contrast to another one [54].

Recently, Harris et al. and Stemkens et al. proposed their similar approaches of 4D-MRI reconstruction based on DIR manipulation and a priori patient-specific motion model [55, 56]. When a 4D-MRI series for a patient is available, a series of DVFs could be generated by DIR. Principal component analysis (PCA) was used to decompose this DVF series into three principle components (PCs). Any future motion imaging could be seen as a simple weighted sum of these three PCs. To derive the three weighting coefficients, the acquisition could be done rapidly by single or multislice 2D acquisition, and the coefficients were solved as a minimization problem based on the similarity of the reconstructed 4D-MRI series at fixed position(s) with 2D acquisition(s) [57]. Because of rapid 2D acquisition, this method could generate volumetric images in cine fashion up to 20 frames/s [57]. Harris et al. also reported that such rapid 2D acquisition can be done by planar KV fluoro images which are widely available on modern radiation linear accelerators

(LINAC) [58, 59]. This point attracts the attention since MR-based radiotherapy treatment guidance can be realized on current radiotherapy platform.

It is crucial to ensure the DIR accuracy when generating the DVF. Li et al. reported their time-resolved 4D-MRI (TR-4DMRI) method with improved DIR reconstruction. Based on the a priori motion information, a pseudo demon force was introduced and applied to the coarse volumetric alignment. The fine-tuning of DIR was performed at multiple resolutions by demon forces [60]. This method was argued with better handle of large anatomy deformation during possible irregular breath. Digital phantom results showed that this technique successfully reconstructed fast 4D series and identified some questionable cases without missing true negative.

The wave of artificial intelligence (AI) in medicine (specifically in radiation oncology imaging) has enlightened many sparkling ideas in medical imaging research [61]. Together with the use of AI in pattern recognition from large-scale data, the currently required patient-specific motion pattern can be potentially derived from population results. Thus, 4D-MRI based on DIR modeling may become the focus of 4D-MRI research in the next decade.

3. 4D-MRI: clinical application

Although 4D-MRI has been demonstrated with great potential of anatomic motion quantification, its application in clinic is still premature for standard practice. Nevertheless, a few works have reported 4D-MRI's values in radiotherapy clinic. In this section, we discuss possible clinical applications of 4D-MRI in radiotherapy.

3.1 Radiotherapy target delineation

Similar to the 4D-CT application, 4D-MRI provides motion direction and quantified motion range information for ITV generation at the same level of accuracy as 4D-CT [62]. Because of superior soft tissue contrast, 4D-MRI may better illustrate ITV definition with finer anatomical detail boundaries.

Figure 5 shows an example of 4D-MRI-based ITV delineation for liver SBRT in our clinic. This case was about liver mets from breast cancer, and the prescription was 16Gy × 3 fractions. 4D-MRI was acquired by bSSFP sequence with 2D-based retrospective sorting [29]. Interslice distance was 5 mm. A total of 10 phase volumes (0, 10, ... 90%) were reconstructed. GTV was contoured in each phase volume as shown by red contours in five representative phase volumes in **Figure 5**. The reference frame of 4D-MRI was registered to the planning CT volume by rigid transform. ITV-MRI, the union of 10 GTVs from 4D-MRI, was mapped to the planning CT as illustrated. The final ITV for this case was adjusted by our radiation oncologist to combine information from both MRI and CT studies.

3.2 Onboard treatment guidance

Since 2010, MR-guided radiotherapy units have become commercially available. The integrated onboard MR imaging capability can provide potentially improved patient positioning accuracy with affluent soft tissue details. In addition, intra-treatment imaging during radiation enables image-based treatment gating, which could reduce margin size for PTV definition with potentially reduced normal tissue toxicity [63]. Currently, both low-field-strength (0.35 T) unit (ViewRay, Oakwood Village, Ohio) and high-field-strength (1.5 T) unit (Elekta AB, Stockholm, Sweden) have started treating patient.

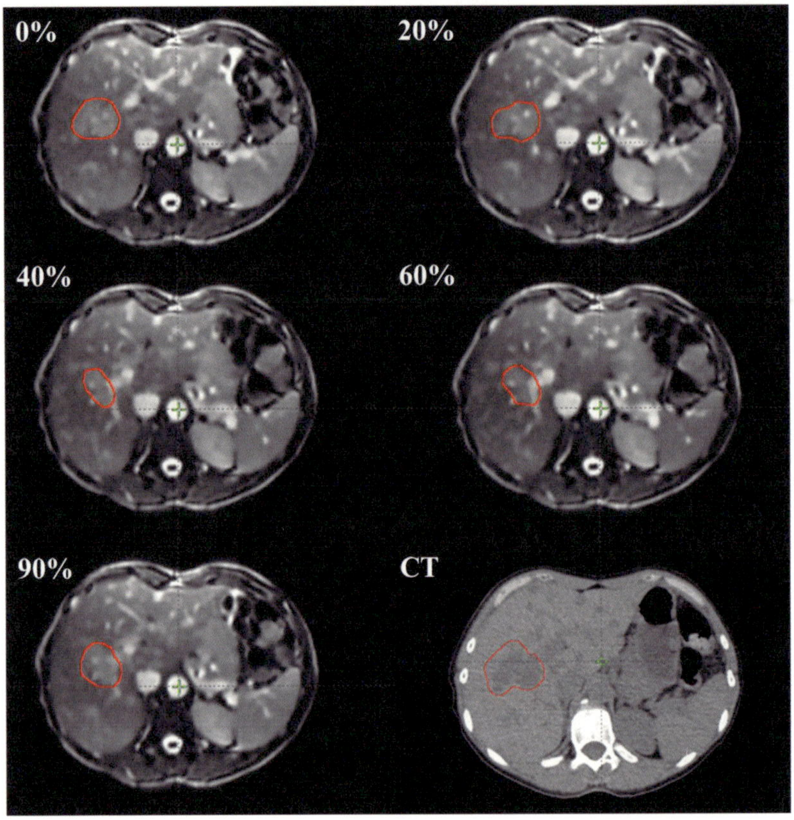

Figure 5.
A clinical example of 4D-MRI in liver SBRT target delineation.

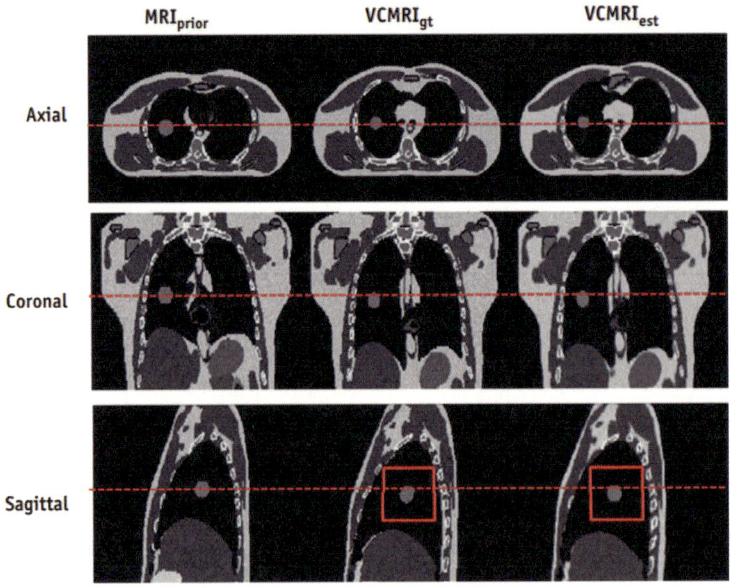

Figure 6.
VC-MRI for onboard MR imaging accuracy simulation. MRI_{prior}, reference EOE volume in pre-treatment 4D-MRI simulation; $VCMRI_{gt}$, ground truth EOI volume at treatment day for onboard match; and $VCMRI_{est}$, estimated EOI volume from the proposed VC-MRI approach.

Onboard image guidance on MR-guided radiotherapy units are implemented by 2D imaging on orthogonal views. Volumetric imaging, though technically feasible, are not realistic because of long imaging time. At this moment, no in vivo implementation of onboard 4D-MRI guidance has been reported. Nevertheless, a few works have tried to demonstrate its feasibility. Harris et al. used digital XCAT phantom simulation to examine their VC-MRI technique for onboard patient positioning accuracy [56]. As shown in **Figure 6**, the estimated VC-MRI volume at end-of-inhalation (EOI) phase (third column) was accurate when comparing to the ground truth volume (second column). The reported target center-of-mass-shift (COMS) was about 1 mm or less on SI direction in most simulation scenarios.

Han et al. implemented their ROCK 4D-MRI technique on their 0.35 T-MR-guided radiotherapy unit [64]. Seven patients with abdominal tumors were imaged with both ROCK 4D-MRI and 2D-cine (reference) techniques. Because of relatively long imaging time (~10 min) in ROCK, image acquisition was performed after treatment as feasibility studies. They reported that when compared with reference 2D-cine results, motion quantification in 4D-MRI was about 1 mm different on SI direction. 3D anatomical details were successfully rendered without motion artifacts for onboard imaging. Optimistically speaking, 4D-MRI for pre-treatment patient positioning could become available in the next decade with novel 4D-MRI methods and improved hardware developments.

Author details

Chunhao Wang* and Fang-Fang Yin
Department of Radiation Oncology, Duke University Medical Center, Durham, NC, United States

*Address all correspondence to: chunhao.wang@duke.edu

References

[1] Khan FM, Gibbons JP. Khan's the Physics of Radiation Therapy. Baltimore, MD: Lippincott Williams & Wilkins; 2014

[2] Landberg T, Chauaudra J, Dobbs H. Prescribing, Recording and Reporting Photon Beam Therapy: ICRU Report 50. Maryland, USA: International Commission on Radiotherapy Units and Measurements; 1993

[3] Ozhasoglu C, Murphy MJ. Issues in respiratory motion compensation during external-beam radiotherapy. International Journal of Radiation Oncology, Biology, Physics. 2002;**52**(5):1389-1399

[4] Stroom JC, Heijmen BJ. Geometrical uncertainties, radiotherapy planning margins, and the ICRU-62 report. Radiotherapy and Oncology. 2002;**64**(1):75-83

[5] Jin J-Y et al. A technique of using gated-CT images to determine internal target volume (ITV) for fractionated stereotactic lung radiotherapy. Radiotherapy and Oncology. 2006;**78**(2):177-184

[6] Siewerdsen J et al. Multimode C-arm fluoroscopy, tomosynthesis, and cone-beam CT for image-guided interventions: From proof of principle to patient protocols. In: Medical Imaging 2007: Physics of Medical Imaging. San Diego, CA: International Society for Optics and Photonics; 2007

[7] Low DA et al. A method for the reconstruction of four-dimensional synchronized CT scans acquired during free breathing. Medical Physics. 2003;**30**(6):1254-1263

[8] Pan T et al. 4D-CT imaging of a volume influenced by respiratory motion on multi-slice CT. Medical Physics. 2004;**31**(2):333-340

[9] Glide-Hurst CK et al. Evaluation of two synchronized external surrogates for 4D CT sorting. Journal of Applied Clinical Medical Physics. 2013;**14**(6):117-132

[10] Quirk S, Becker N, Smith W. External respiratory motion analysis and statistics for patients and volunteers. Journal of Applied Clinical Medical Physics. 2013;**14**(2):90-101

[11] Hoisak JD et al. Correlation of lung tumor motion with external surrogate indicators of respiration. International Journal of Radiation Oncology, Biology, Physics. 2004;**60**(4):1298-1306

[12] Ruan D et al. Inference of hysteretic respiratory tumor motion from external surrogates: A state augmentation approach. Physics in Medicine & Biology. 2008;**53**(11):2923

[13] Lattanzi J et al. Ultrasound-based stereotactic guidance of precision conformal external beam radiation therapy in clinically localized prostate cancer. Urology. 2000;**55**(1):73-78

[14] Fuss M et al. Daily ultrasound-based image-guided targeting for radiotherapy of upper abdominal malignancies. International Journal of Radiation Oncology, Biology, Physics. 2004;**59**(4):1245-1256

[15] O'shea T, Bamber J, Harris E. MO-DE-210-05: Improved accuracy of liver feature motion estimation in B-Mode ultrasound for image-guided radiation therapy. Medical Physics. 2015;**42**(6Part28):3560-3560

[16] Mason SA et al. Towards ultrasound-guided adaptive radiotherapy for cervical cancer:

Evaluation of Elekta's semiautomated uterine segmentation method on 3D ultrasound images. Medical Physics. 2017;**44**(7):3630-3638

[17] Dawson LA, Sharpe MB. Image-guided radiotherapy: Rationale, benefits, and limitations. The Lancet Oncology. 2006;**7**(10):848-858

[18] Koch N et al. Evaluation of internal lung motion for respiratory-gated radiotherapy using MRI: Part I—correlating internal lung motion with skin fiducial motion. International Journal of Radiation Oncology, Biology, Physics. 2004;**60**(5):1459-1472

[19] Shimizu S et al. High-speed magnetic resonance imaging for four-dimensional treatment planning of conformal radiotherapy of moving body tumors1. International Journal of Radiation Oncology, Biology, Physics. 2000;**48**(2):471-474

[20] Kirilova A et al. Three-dimensional motion of liver tumors using cine-magnetic resonance imaging. International Journal of Radiation Oncology, Biology, Physics. 2008;**71**(4):1189-1195

[21] Feng M et al. Characterization of pancreatic tumor motion using cine MRI: Surrogates for tumor position should be used with caution. International Journal of Radiation Oncology, Biology, Physics. 2009;**74**(3):884-891

[22] Cai J et al. Evaluation of the reproducibility of lung motion probability distribution function (PDF) using dynamic MRI. Physics in Medicine & Biology. 2006;**52**(2):365

[23] Blackall J et al. MRI-based measurements of respiratory motion variability and assessment of imaging strategies for radiotherapy planning. Physics in Medicine & Biology. 2006;**51**(17):4147

[24] Dinkel J et al. 4D-MRI analysis of lung tumor motion in patients with hemidiaphragmatic paralysis. Radiotherapy and Oncology. 2009;**91**(3):449-454

[25] Tryggestad E et al. Respiration-based sorting of dynamic MRI to derive representative 4D-MRI for radiotherapy planning. Medical Physics. 2013;**40**(5):051909

[26] von Siebenthal M et al. 4D MR imaging of respiratory organ motion and its variability. Physics in Medicine & Biology. 2007;**52**(6):1547

[27] Remmert G et al. Four-dimensional magnetic resonance imaging for the determination of tumour movement and its evaluation using a dynamic porcine lung phantom. Physics in Medicine & Biology. 2007;**52**(18):N401

[28] Hu Y et al. Respiratory amplitude guided 4-dimensional magnetic resonance imaging. International Journal of Radiation Oncology Biology Physics. 2013;**86**(1):198-204

[29] Cai J et al. Four-dimensional magnetic resonance imaging (4D-MRI) using image-based respiratory surrogate: A feasibility study. Medical Physics. 2011;**38**(12):6384-6394

[30] Tokuda J et al. Adaptive 4D MR imaging using navigator-based respiratory signal for MRI-guided therapy. Magnetic Resonance in Medicine. 2008;**59**(5):1051-1061

[31] Deng Z et al. Four-dimensional MRI using three-dimensional radial sampling with respiratory self-gating to characterize temporal phase-resolved respiratory motion in the abdomen. Magnetic Resonance in Medicine. 2016;**75**(4):1574-1585

[32] Pang J et al. Accelerated whole-heart coronary MRA using motion-corrected

sensitivity encoding with three-dimensional projection reconstruction. Magnetic Resonance in Medicine. 2015;**73**(1):284-291

[33] Feng L et al. XD-GRASP: Golden-angle radial MRI with reconstruction of extra motion-state dimensions using compressed sensing. Magnetic Resonance in Medicine. 2016;**75**(2):775-788

[34] Han F et al. Respiratory motion-resolved, self-gated 4D-MRI using rotating cartesian k-space (ROCK). Medical Physics. 2017;**44**(4):1359-1368

[35] Wang C et al. A spatiotemporal-constrained sorting method for motion-robust 4D-MRI: A feasibility study. International Journal of Radiation Oncology, Biology, Physics. 2018;**103**(3):758-766

[36] Kazantsev IG, Matej S, Lewitt RM. Optimal ordering of projections using permutation matrices and angles between projection subspaces. Electronic Notes in Discrete Mathematics. 2005;**20**:205-216

[37] Tsai CM, Nishimura DG. Reduced aliasing artifacts using variable-density k-space sampling trajectories. Magnetic Resonance in Medicine. 2000;**43**(3):452-458

[38] Chan RW et al. Temporal stability of adaptive 3D radial MRI using multidimensional golden means. Magnetic Resonance in Medicine. 2009;**61**(2):354-363

[39] Pang J et al. ECG and navigator-free four-dimensional whole-heart coronary MRA for simultaneous visualization of cardiac anatomy and function. Magnetic Resonance in Medicine. 2014;**72**(5):1208-1217

[40] Jiang SB. Technical aspects of image-guided respiration-gated radiation therapy. Medical Dosimetry. 2006;**31**(2):141-151

[41] Lu W et al. A comparison between amplitude sorting and phase-angle sorting using external respiratory measurement for 4D CT. Medical Physics. 2006;**33**(8):2964-2974

[42] Cheng JY et al. Free-breathing pediatric MRI with nonrigid motion correction and acceleration. Journal of Magnetic Resonance Imaging. 2015;**42**(2):407-420

[43] Uecker M et al. ESPIRiT—an eigenvalue approach to autocalibrating parallel MRI: Where SENSE meets GRAPPA. Magnetic Resonance in Medicine. 2014;**71**(3):990-1001

[44] Gamper U, Boesiger P, Kozerke S. Compressed sensing in dynamic MRI. Magnetic Resonance in Medicine. 2008;**59**(2):365-373

[45] Lustig M, Donoho D, Pauly JM. Sparse MRI: The application of compressed sensing for rapid MR imaging. Magnetic Resonance in Medicine. 2007;**58**(6):1182-1195

[46] Donoho DL. Compressed sensing. IEEE Transactions on Information Theory. 2006;**52**(4):1289-1306

[47] Block KT, Uecker M, Frahm J. Undersampled radial MRI with multiple coils. Iterative image reconstruction using a total variation constraint. Magnetic Resonance in Medicine. 2007;**57**(6):1086-1098

[48] Knoll F et al. Second order total generalized variation (TGV) for MRI. Magnetic Resonance in Medicine. 2011;**65**(2):480-491

[49] Ying L, Xu D, Liang Z-P. On Tikhonov regularization for image reconstruction in parallel MRI. In: Engineering in Medicine and Biology Society, 2004. IEMBS'04. 26th Annual International Conference of the IEEE. IEEE; 2004

[50] Daubechies I, Defrise M, De Mol C. An iterative thresholding algorithm for linear inverse problems with a sparsity constraint. Communications on Pure and Applied Mathematics. 2004;**57**(11):1413-1457

[51] Wang C et al. Accelerated brain DCE-MRI using iterative reconstruction with total generalized variation penalty for quantitative pharmacokinetic analysis: A feasibility study. Technology in Cancer Research & Treatment. 2017;**16**(4):446-460

[52] Subashi E et al. A comparison of radial keyhole strategies for high spatial and temporal resolution 4D contrast-enhanced MRI in small animal tumor models. Medical Physics. 2013;**40**(2):022304

[53] Brock KK, Consortium DRA. Results of a multi-institution deformable registration accuracy study (MIDRAS). International Journal of Radiation Oncology, Biology, Physics. 2010;**76**(2):583-596

[54] Yang J et al. Four-dimensional magnetic resonance imaging using axial body area as respiratory surrogate: Initial patient results. International Journal of Radiation Oncology, Biology, Physics. 2014;**88**(4):907-912

[55] Stemkens B et al. Image-driven, model-based 3D abdominal motion estimation for MR-guided radiotherapy. Physics in Medicine & Biology. 2016;**61**(14):5335

[56] Harris W et al. A technique for generating volumetric cine-magnetic resonance imaging. International Journal of Radiation Oncology, Biology, Physics. 2016;**95**(2):844-853

[57] Wang C et al. TU-AB-BRA-09: A novel method of generating ultrafast volumetric cine MRI (VC-MRI) using prior 4D-MRI and on-board phase-skipped encoding acquisition for radiotherapy target localization. Medical Physics. 2016;**43**(6Part33):3735-3735

[58] Wang C et al. A novel method of generating onboard 4D-MRI for liver SBRT target localization using prior 4D-MRI simulation and onboard limited angle kV acquisition from a conventional LINAC. International Journal of Radiation Oncology Biology Physics. 2017;**99**(2):S126-S127

[59] Harris W et al. A novel method to generate on-board 4D MRI using prior 4D MRI and on-board kV projections from a conventional LINAC for target localization in liver SBRT. Medical Physics. 2018;**45**(7):3238-3245

[60] Li G et al. Introduction of a pseudo demons force to enhance deformation range for robust reconstruction of super-resolution time-resolved 4 DMRI. Medical Physics. 2018;**45**(11):5197-5207

[61] Thompson RF et al. Artificial intelligence in radiation oncology imaging. International Journal of Radiation Oncology Biology Physics. 2018;**102**(4):1159-1161

[62] Oar A et al. Comparison of four dimensional computed tomography and magnetic resonance imaging in abdominal radiotherapy planning. Physics and Imaging in Radiation Oncology. 2018;**7**:70-75

[63] Lagendijk JJ, Raaymakers BW, Van Vulpen M. The magnetic resonance imaging–linac system. Seminars in Radiation Oncology. Philadelphia, PA: WB Saunders; 2014;**24**(3)

[64] Han F et al. Respiratory motion-resolved, self-gated 4D-MRI using rotating Cartesian K-space (ROCK): Initial clinical experience on an MRI-guided radiotherapy system. Radiotherapy and Oncology. 2018;**127**(3):467-473